your guide to

bowel
cancer

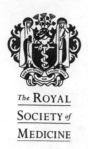

The ROYAL
SOCIETY *of*
MEDICINE

your guide to

bowel
cancer

Professor John Northover
Dr Joel Kettner
Mr Barry Paraskeva

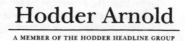

Hodder Arnold

A MEMBER OF THE HODDER HEADLINE GROUP

Orders: Please contact Bookpoint Ltd, 130 Milton Park,
Abingdon, Oxon OX14 4SB. Telephone: (44) 01235 827720,
Fax: (44) 01235 400454. Lines are open from 9.00 to
17.00, Monday to Saturday, with a 24-hour message
answering service. You can also order through our website
www.hoddereducation.com

British Library Cataloguing in Publication Data
A catalogue record for this title is available from the British
Library.

ISBN-10: 0 340 927461
ISBN-13: 9 780340 927465

First published   2007
Impression number   10 9 8 7 6 5 4 3 2 1
Year   2010   2009   2008   2007

Typeset by Servis Filmsetting Limited, Longsight, Manchester.
Printed in Great Britain for Hodder Arnold, a division of
Hodder Headline, 338 Euston Road, London NW1 3BH,
by Cox & Wyman Ltd, Reading, Berkshire.

Hodder Headline's policy is to use papers that are natural,
renewable and recyclable products and made from wood
grown in sustainable forests. The logging and manufacturing
processes are expected to conform to the environmental
regulations of the country of origin.

Every effort has been made to trace copyright for material used
in this book. The authors and publishers would be happy to
make arrangements with any holder of copyright whom it has
not been possible to trace successfully by the time of going to
press.

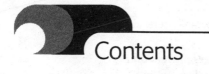

Contents

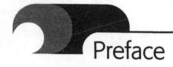

Preface

This new book, published in partnership with the Royal Society of Medicine, provides detailed, useful and up-to-date information on bowel cancer. It contains expert yet user-friendly advice, with such useful features as:

Key terms: demystifying the jargon
Questions and Answers: answering the burning questions
Myths and Facts: debunking the misconceptions
My Experience: how it feels to live with, or care for someone with, this condition.

Bearing the hallmark of excellence and accessibility that characterizes the work of the Royal Society of Medicine, this important guide will enable you and your family to gain some control over the way your bowel cancer is managed by being better informed.

Peter Richardson
Director of Publications
Royal Society of Medicine

While every effort has been made to ensure that the contents of this book are as accurate and up to date as possible, neither the publishers nor the authors can be held responsible for errors or for any consequences arising from the use of information contained herein.

Do not attempt to self-diagnose or self-treat for any serious or long-term problems – always seek advice first from a medical professional or qualified practitioner.*

Foreword

Many people recall the iconic photographs and film footage of Bobby Moore holding the Jules Rimet Trophy aloft on that glorious sunny day at Wembley in July 1966 when England won the World Cup. What they don't know is that he died far too young of a highly curable disease; bowel cancer.

As an ex-professional footballer and athlete, a disciplined man who maintained a high level of fitness even into his forties, Bobby knew immediately that there was something physically wrong. He was 46 and had rectal bleeding, was visiting the lavatory four or five times a night when previously he would only go once every morning.

We did not know it back then in 1986, but these were clear high risk bowel cancer symptoms and needed to be checked out. We did however, despite our ignorance, immediately seek advice from our local GP who, during that same week arranged for us to visit a Harley Street specialist. The specialist told Bobby that he had a condition called Irritable Bowel Syndrome, which was not life threatening and advised that Bobby should go away and live life normally. Naturally Bobby was relieved.

At this time we moved to another area and, because the symptoms persisted, we again sought help from our new doctor who confirmed the specialist's findings. Bobby persisted in returning to his GP every few months only to be told that this condition, IBS, though incurable, was not sinister. Just prior to Bobby's 50th birthday, in desperation, Bobby asked to see another specialist.

Within the week Bobby had been diagnosed with bowel cancer, followed by an operation to remove a malignant tumour from his colon. The operation had been a success. The tumour had been removed and no colostomy was required but secondary metastasizes had been sighted on both lobes of his liver. This was to prove fatal. Bobby's condition was not curable, though the chemotherapy and the radiotherapy would buy Bobby some more time. He died at home, aged just 51, of a disease, which if diagnosed early, is over 90% curable.

Bowel cancer still claims more lives in the UK than any other cancer except lung cancer and yet it remains an unspoken about disease.

After Bobby died, I decided to do all in my power to help to change these desperate statistics. I founded a charity in Bobby's name, which raises much needed funds for dedicated bowel cancer research and strives to enlighten the public about the disease and its high risk symptoms.

Now, there are clear guidelines for GPs on the symptoms that require an urgent referral to a specialist. Treatment for bowel cancer is far more sophisticated than it was in 1991 when Bobby's condition was finally diagnosed and bowel cancer statistics are improving all the time. More people are being diagnosed with bowel cancer and more people are being successfully treated than ever before.

This book dispels all the mystery surrounding the medical terms used when describing bowel cancer and I have found it most useful. If this book had been available to us in 1986 when Bobby first tried to seek help, he probably would be alive today. I would have a husband, his children, a father and his grandchildren, a grandfather. If you want to know as much as possible about bowel cancer, I would recommend this book.

Stephanie Moore MBE
Founder of the Bobby Moore Fund
for Cancer Research UK

Introduction

Bowel cancer is primarily a disease of the industrially developed world, and it is one of the inevitable hazards for countries moving towards the so-called Western lifestyle. Throughout Europe, North America and Australasia this is one of the 'big three' cancers; in the UK around one person in 20 will get bowel cancer and one in 50 will die from it.

Yet even during the careers of the authors, so much has changed, and there is every reason to think that these favourable trends will gain more momentum. However, for now we must consider the significance of the disease today, how it impacts on the lives of patients and their families and what we can offer to prevent and to mitigate the consequences of this common disease.

There is no doubt that in the past 25 years, bowel cancer has been confronted more realistically by individuals, by society and by successive governments. People are becoming more aware of the symptoms of bowel cancer and are less reluctant to come forward for advice and for treatment if the diagnosis is made. Surgery has become a much more specialist exercise, with an added emphasis on delicacy and precision in the complex procedures involved. The methods of investigation have changed almost beyond recognition in a generation, allowing much more informed decision-making in the types and combinations of treatment methods. The range of treatments has widened considerably, and in particular the armamentarium of the medical oncologist has been strengthened, even over the past ten years. Perhaps the most important strategic development in decades has been the recent implementation of population screening in the UK, based on 30 years of painstaking scientific research, which is destined to cut the death rate by 15 to 20 per cent when implemented fully across the population.

We have witnessed the growth of the holistic approach during the past 25 years, with much more attention to the patient rather than just to the disease. As part of this there has been the exponential expansion in the role of the specialist nurses, who have taken their experience and expertise in the time-honoured and fundamental role at the bedside and applied it in such vital fields as stoma care, oncology and endoscopy. There is also the emergence of the clinical nurse specialist, who so often these days coordinates care across the whole range and offers empathy and practical support to each new patient facing the challenges of diagnosis and treatment.

Knowledge forearms, while lack of it engenders fear. In this book we aim to give some insight into what bowel cancer is, how it comes about, how it behaves and how it can be dealt with effectively. We try to explain how modern methods allow doctors, nurses and patients to apply to best effect the wide range of powerful tools now available. We also look at the prospects for even more effective care in the future as the full panoply of clinical and laboratory research improves our understanding and therefore our ability to challenge this important disease.

CHAPTER

1

The bowel: what it is and what it does

This book will look in detail at how bowel cancer develops, what symptoms it may cause and how it can be treated. To understand these subjects it helps to understand the normal anatomy and physiology of the bowel – where and what it is and how it works. As we go through this basic description, we will introduce many of the technical terms it will be necessary to know.

The word **bowel** is derived from the Latin word *botellus* (meaning 'sausage'). The bowel is a very long tube, longer than the average family laid head to toe – in which the food we eat is digested and absorbed, what is left being returned to the outside world as **faeces** and flatus ('wind'). The bowel consists of two main parts, the 'small' and 'large' bowels. When we talk of bowel cancer, however, we are referring to the **large bowel** – cancer of the **small bowel** is rare, and will not be covered here. The small bowel is about four times the length of the large

bowel
A 4–6 metre muscular tube within which food is digested and the 'goodness' absorbed, and from which the remainder is expelled.

faeces
Solid part of waste expelled via anus (sometimes called 'stool', especially by doctors and nurses).

large bowel
A 1–1.5 metre section where 80 per cent of water is absorbed, leaving faeces for explusion.

small bowel
A 4 metre section where food is digested and useful parts absorbed.

colon

First and longest part of large bowel, where water is absorbed.

rectum

Last 15 cm of large bowel, where faeces are stored before expulsion.

anal canal

A 4 cm tube between the rectum and anus, surrounded by sphincter muscles that control expulsion.

anus

Opening from anal canal to the outside world.

anal cancer

Rare cancer arising from skin of anal canal or anus (300 cases a year in UK compared to 35,000 cases of colorectal cancer).

gastrointestinal tract (GIT)

Whole length of tube, from mouth to anus, where food is processed to provide energy and building materials for body tissues.

bowel (it is the greater width of the large bowel that accounts for its name). Other names for the large bowel are the large intestine, and the **colon** and **rectum** – hence bowel cancer may also be called colorectal cancer. The rectum is often considered as the final passageway to the outside world, but that distinction belongs to the **anal canal**, the last four centimetres of the digestive tract, leading to the external opening, the **anus**. The anal canal is not technically part of the rectum and therefore is not usually considered as part of the large bowel. **Anal cancer** – even more rare than cancer of the small bowel – is a different cancer yet again and will not be dealt with in this book. However, because of the relevance of the anal canal to the workings of the large bowel, and to the surgical treatment of bowel cancer, its anatomy and function will be described in this chapter.

What is the large bowel?

Only about five to ten percent of the volume of the food we eat finds its way to the large bowel (and eventually out of it!) after passing through the oral cavity (mouth), the pharynx (throat), the oesophagus (gullet or foodpipe), the stomach, and the small bowel. The large bowel is about 1.5 metres in lengh. The whole system, from mouth to anus, is called the **gastrointestinal tract (GIT)**.

The main function of those parts of the GIT that have handled the food before it gets to the colon is to break it down by physical and chemical means. This allows the useful components of food to be absorbed (mainly by the small bowel) into the bloodstream, by which it is taken to the liver and then to all parts of the body to be used as a source of energy, for growth and repair. By the time the remaining material reaches the large bowel, pretty much anything nutritious has been absorbed. This undigested material is no longer sterile (i.e. free of bacteria, as it was in the stomach and upper part of the small bowel) but is now heavily loaded with the bacteria that normally inhabit the bowel to aid digestion; the major proportion of faeces comprises dead bacteria and bowel wall cells, shed routinely at the end of their short lives.

The colon, rectum, and anal canal perform several vital tasks. They:

✧ absorb water from the intestinal contents – this decreases the volume by around 80 per cent
✧ lubricate and propel the faeces
✧ store the faeces and flatus
✧ finally evacuate them from the body.

The colon absorbs and propels, the rectum stores and 'evacuates' via the anal canal.

Development of the bowel

It is worth spending a little while thinking about just how the bowel develops in the embryo because this helps us to understand how it works in the adult.

When the embryo is just a few millimetres long, a straight hollow tube called the primitive gut has already formed. Soon this grows into the beginnings of the series of organs that makes up the adult GIT. As it develops, three areas, the 'foregut', the 'midgut', and the 'hindgut' (from which the stomach and intestine grow) can be

Q So why don't we already know most of this?

A For many people discussion of bowels, especially what they do, is embarrassing or even impolite – hence most are not very aware of bowel cancer. In many societies this taboo is not seen, and in some countries they even design the lavatories to help people inspect their 'poo'!

recognized, each with its own blood and nerve supplies; each segment has its own major artery from the body's main artery (the aorta), each breaking up into many branches. The foregut has the coeliac (pronounced 'seal-ee-ack') artery, the midgut has the superior mesenteric artery, and the hindgut has the inferior mesenteric artery ('superior' and 'inferior' in this context mean 'upper' and 'lower'). Each artery has corresponding veins, as well as lymphatic vessels, which take body fluid from the intestinal tissues back to the blood stream. These lymphatic vessels are very important in the spread of cancer.

The abdominal cavity

The bowels and the other digestive organs lie in the **abdominal cavity**, which stretches from as high as the level of the nipples down to the pelvis. It is lined by a membrane called the **peritoneum**. The bowels are packed into part of this space; some parts can move around to some extent, while other organs, such as the liver and some parts of the large bowel, are held in position.

Digestion and the general arrangement of organs

Food passes down the oesophagus and into the stomach where digestion begins (see Figure 1.1). Then the partially digested food passes into the **duodenum**, in the centre of the upper abdomen. The liver and pancreas, both situated in the upper abdomen, deliver digestive juices to the duodenum. The food then enters the small

abdominal cavity
Area within the abdomen containing the intestine, liver, uterus, bladder and other abdominal organs.

peritoneum
Inner lining of the abdominal cavity.

myth
'Stomach' is just another word for 'abdomen'.

fact
When people think this, they can mistake 'stomach cancer' for 'bowel cancer', two very different diseases.

duodenum
The first 12 cm of the bowel beyond the stomach, where important digestive juices enter from the liver and pancreas.

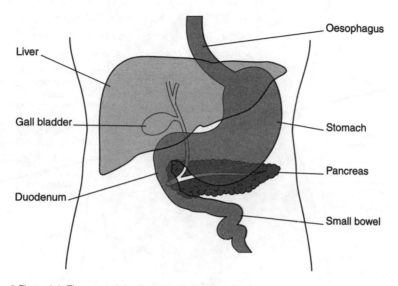

Figure 1.1 The upper abdominal digestive organs. Food reaches the stomach via the oesophagus (gullet). Acid digestion begins in the stomach, after which food passes into the duodenum where bile and pancreatic 'juice' are added, prior to entry into the upper small bowel, where digestion is completed and absorption begins.

bowel, which is around four metres long, coiled in the central abdomen, and free to move as it churns the digested food to aid its absorption. The small bowel is attached to the back of the abdominal cavity by a sheet of tissue called the **mesentery** – through this run the arteries, veins, lymphatics and nerves to the bowel.

The colon is generally more fixed in position than the small bowel, and it looks very different (see Figure 1.2). Whereas the small bowel is a smooth tube, around three to four centimetres wide, the colon is wider (five to seven centimetres), looks rather crumpled, and has

mesentery
Sheet of tissue attaching the small bowel to the back of the abdominal cavity, carrying arteries and veins to the bowel from the body's main blood vessels (aorta and vena cava).

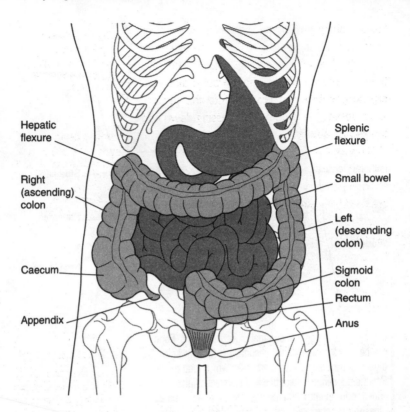

Figure 1.2 The colon, rectum and anus. The small bowel empties into the first part of the colon, the caecum. This fluid, containing the leftovers of digestion, is transported through the colon, where most of the water is reabsorbed into the bloodstream. The remainder, i.e. the faeces, are held temporarily in the rectum prior to voiding at a convenient time.

caecum
First part of the colon, lying in right, lower abdomen. Small bowel empties into it.

appendix
Worm-like, blind-ending tube, several centimetres long. Best known as the site of appendicitis, and can rarely give rise to cancer.

three one centimetre strips of muscle (taeniae) running along it throughout, which helps surgeons distinguish the colon from the small bowel. The colon begins in the right lower abdomen as the **caecum** (pronounced 'see-cum'); the **appendix** is attached to the caecum. After this the colon runs up the right side of the abdomen (the right, or ascending, colon); next it takes a sharp turn to the left across the upper abdomen (transverse colon), and then down the left side (left, or descending, colon). After this there is a section that can move around called the **sigmoid colon** that empties into the rectum, which leaves the abdomen by passing down into the **pelvic cavity**.

Although the colon is mobile to some extent, it is not entirely free to flop around in the abdominal cavity since its right and left portions are fixed fairly firmly to the back of the abdominal cavity. In contrast, the transverse colon and sigmoid colon are more mobile because each has a mesentery, like the small bowel.

As pointed out earlier, the large bowel is divided into the colon and rectum by anatomists; each has special functions.

Finer points of colonic anatomy

Blood circulation

After the blood has passed through the lungs to collect oxygen, the heart pumps it into the body's largest artery, the aorta, which runs down from the chest into the abdominal cavity. Large branches go to each of the important organs including the bowel, each branch giving further branches, and so on, ending as microscopically small blood vessels, the capillaries. These allow the release of oxygen to, and absorption of digested food and water from, the bowel (see Figure 1.3). The blood is then collected in veins which join up, ultimately to form the **portal vein**, which passes into the liver, where much of its nutritious content is removed and stored. The blood then returns to the heart and lungs to be

sigmoid colon
Last part of colon before the rectum and the commonest site for colon cancer.

pelvic cavity
Area immediately below abdominal cavity, surrounded by bony pelvis, and mainly containing rectum, bladder and uterus.

myth
Circulation is simple: blood just goes from the heart to the whole body in the arteries and comes back in the veins.

fact
The gastrointestinal tract has its own special vein (the portal vein), which takes all its blood to the liver to drop off food and to pick up energy supplies before the blood returns to the heart.

portal vein
Large vein that drains all the blood away from the bowel, and carries it to the liver.

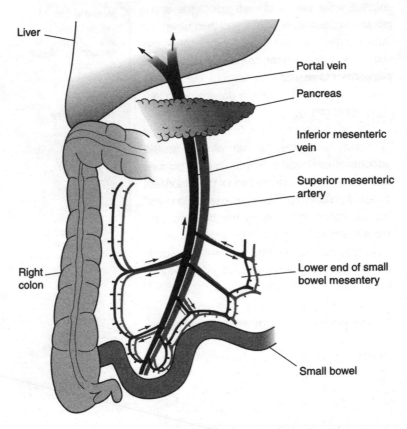

Figure 1.3 Blood supply to the intestines. Blood passes to the small bowel and right colon via the superior mesenteric artery; after delivering oxygen and collecting digested food, the blood travels to the liver via the superior mesenteric and portal veins. The rest of the colon and rectum (not shown here) receive blood via the inferior mesenteric artery; the inferior mesenteric vein drains into the portal vein. Cancer cells that have become detached from bowel tumours can reach the liver by being carried in the mesenteric and portal veins.

pumped around again. If a cancer is growing in the bowel, cancer cells may get into the blood stream within the bowel wall, and can thereby reach the liver, where they can grow into **secondary tumours**.

Lymph circulation

The lymph circulation is part of the body's defence system. Its other function is to collect the fluid that has been released from the capillaries to deliver oxygen and 'food' to each and every body cell, and then return that fluid to the bloodstream. The **lymphatic circulation** is made up of a massive network of very thin walled tubes that run with the arteries and veins carrying blood to and from all parts (Figure 1.4). In cancer patients, the lymphatic vessels may also pick up malignant cells that have escaped from the tumour, giving them access to the rest of the body. Along these lymphatic channels, which run next to the corresponding arteries, are lymph glands (sometimes called 'lymph nodes'), rather like stations along a railway line. There are thousands of these glands in the body and they produce lymphocytes, which are cells that attack bacteria (germs) and other cells (including those escaping from primary cancers) recognized by them as foreign to the body.

The lymphocytes and other defence cells may be quite important in the body's ability to deal with cancer, but unfortunately they seem not to always function well in this role. Sometimes cancer cells can overwhelm the defences and grow into secondary tumours in the lymph glands, from where they can spread onwards into the bloodstream. In this way tumour cells get to

secondary tumours
Islands of cancer widely separated from the original ('primary') tumour in the colon or rectum. Can grow anywhere in the body, but the liver is the commonest site. They start from cancer cells escaping from the primary, and are carried elsewhere in the blood (initially via the portal vein).

lymphatic circulation
System of fine tubes and glands found throughout the body. Some of the body's defence cells (lymphocytes) are produced in the glands. Cancer cells escaping from the primary cancer can travel in lymph vessels and settle in the lymph glands, and grow into secondary tumours.

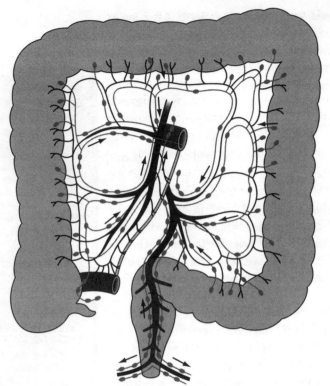

Figure 1.4 Lymphatic drainage of the large bowel. Tissue fluid ('lymph') drains from the bowel wall into microscopic lymph channels, and onwards to the lymph glands. (The lymph glands are shown as grey dots and the direction of lymph flow by arrows.) Besides ultimately draining lymph back into the bloodstream, the lymphatic channels may carry cancer cells to the lymph glands and onwards to the bloodstream.

other parts of the body, where they may settle and grow. The presence or absence of clumps of tumour cells in the lymph glands is an important sign to the pathologist trying to estimate the chance of cure offered by the surgery. This will be discussed later in the book.

Anatomy of the rectum and anal canal

The word rectum is derived from the Latin *rectus*, which means 'straight'. The rectum begins as the sigmoid colon ends – at the **rectosigmoid junction** – and passes downwards through the pelvis to reach the upper end of the anal canal. The upper half of the rectum lies in the abdominal cavity and the lower half in the pelvis. Immediately behind the rectum is the sacrum (the bone of the low back, which can be felt between the upper parts of the buttocks), and the coccyx ('tailbone'). Sometimes rectal tumours spread backwards to involve the sacrum and the nerves to the pelvis and legs that emerge through it – this can cause very severe pain.

Some very important structures lie in front of the rectum (see Figure 1.5). In men these are, from below upwards, the **prostate** and seminal vesicles (which together produce semen), the vasa deferentia (which carry sperm from the testicles to the prostate and **urethra** and are tied and cut in vasectomy), the **ureters**, and the urinary bladder itself. In women, the **uterus** lies in front of the upper part of the rectum and the back wall of the vagina lies immediately in front of the lower rectum. The **ovaries**, **Fallopian tubes** and, in both sexes, some of the small bowel lie around the upper part of the rectum, within the abdominal cavity. The close relationship to the rectum of these important organs poses extra problems for the surgeon in deciding how to tackle some rectal cancers – any of these organs can be invaded by a growing rectal cancer, and so may have to be removed if cure is to be attempted.

rectosigmoid junction
Point in the upper pelvic cavity where the sigmoid colon empties into the top of the rectum.

prostate
Chestnut-sized organ, found only in men, lying just below the bladder. It produces some of the material that goes to make up the semen.

urethra
Tube from bladder through which urine leaves the body. Longer in the male as it passes through the penis.

ureters
Tubes that carry urine from the kidneys to the bladder.

uterus
A 7–8 cm pear-shaped muscular organ within which eggs are fertilized, and the resulting foetus grows into a baby.

ovaries
Female organs, about the shape and size of a flattened cherry, where eggs ('ova') are produced for reproduction.

Fallopian tubes
Two tubes, each running from an ovary to the uterus, whose job it is to capture released eggs, and carry them to the uterus for possible fertilization.

(a)

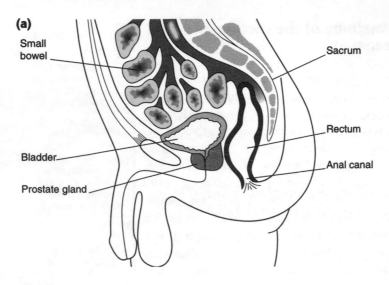

Small bowel

Sacrum

Rectum

Anal canal

Bladder

Prostate gland

(b)

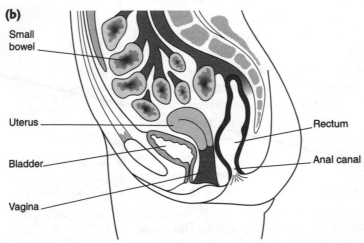

Small bowel

Uterus

Rectum

Bladder

Anal canal

Vagina

Figure 1.5 Important structures in front of the rectum. (a) Male – The small bowel, within the peritoneal cavity, lies in front of the upper rectum. Below the peritoneal cavity the bladder and prostate are immediately in front of the rectum. (b) Female – The upper rectum has the small bowel in front of it, while the uterus and vagina lie in front of the lower half.

The anal canal, which is about 4 cm (1½ inches) long, is a complex structure with important and delicate tasks. It is the outlet from the rectum and is surrounded by the anal sphincter muscles, which maintain continence by staying constantly contracted while allowing defaecation by a reflex that makes the muscles relax.

Blood supply, lymphatics and nerves of the rectum and anal canal

The rectum and anal canal receive their blood mainly from two arteries: the inferior mesenteric and internal iliac arteries. Blood returns from the rectum to the circulation, like the rest of the blood from the bowel, via the portal vein to the liver.

The lymph vessels from the rectum travel alongside the blood vessels and proceed in two directions:

✧ upwards – accompanying the inferior mesenteric vessels and draining into the glands around the aorta
✧ laterally (i.e. sideways) – travelling to the lymph glands around the internal iliac arteries on each side wall of the pelvis.

Like those supplying the colon, the nerves of the rectum are part of the **autonomic nervous system**. The rectum is sensitive to pressure and stretching – these nerves make us aware of whether it is distended with faeces and/or flatus and hence in need of emptying.

autonomic nervous system
The system of nerves throughout the body that mediate control of many of the body's routine functions, like the beating of the heart, muscular action of the bowel, dilatation and contraction of blood vessels. These nerves cannot be 'fired' at will, so for instance, we cannot consciously alter our heart rate.

Nerves supplying organs around the rectum

The urinary and reproductive organs also receive their nerve supply from the autonomic system. They tell us when the bladder needs emptying and control the muscles that achieve this. They also control penile erection and ejaculation of semen. Sometimes any or all of these nerves may be severed during surgery for rectal cancer, as extensive removal of tissues around the rectum may be necessary to get the best chance of cure. The consequences of surgical interference with these nerves will be discussed later.

Down the microscope

The appearance of the bowel seen down a microscope reflects its functions. It is organized into two parts: the inner lining ('**mucosa**', aka 'epithelium') and the outer wall (muscle tube).

The inner lining of the bowel – the mucosa

The inner lining of the large bowel is in contact with the faeces; it is from these cells that bowel cancer develops. The epithelial cells are fast-growing; normally they have a very short life before they are shed into the faeces and replaced by new ones. This feature of rapid growth and turnover may be a factor in the susceptibility of the bowel to developing cancer. It is also the reason why the bowel and other parts of the gut are so sensitive to agents that can damage growing and reproducing cells, such as radiation and cancer-killing drugs. Destruction of the

mucosa
The tissue lining the inside of the small and large bowel, in some areas producing some of the chemicals to digest food, and in others absorbing the products of digestion and water left over from the process. It also produces mucus (hence its name), which protects the mucosa and lubricates the passage of faeces.

epithelial lining of the gut is one of the prominent features of radiation sickness (from nuclear blasts and accidents), and is one of the reasons for side effects from cancer treatments employing drugs or radiation.

The outer layer of the bowel wall – the muscle layer

The bowel has two outer layers of muscle, which propel its contents onwards. The nerves that control it work independently of conscious control.

What does the large bowel do?

The colon

The colon serves two main functions: recovery of water from its contents, and propulsion of the resulting faeces to the rectum for timely evacuation.

Absorption of fluid

About one litre of intestinal fluid reaches the colon every day from the small bowel. Of this, normally only about one-fifth is passed as faeces, while the remainder is re-absorbed into the bloodstream. Loss of this absorptive capacity (whether due to disease or surgical removal) can cause severe diarrhoea.

Propulsion of faeces

While absorbing fluid, the colon also propels its contents onwards. This occurs more slowly than in the small bowel – the intestinal content reaches the colon about four or five hours after swallowing, but it takes two or three times as long to get around the colon and rectum. Thus 24 hours is the average time for completion of the journey through the entire digestive tract.

The rectum and anal canal

Despite their important functions, the rectum and anal canal, like the colon, are not vital or essential organs – in other words, we can if necessary live without them. Two hundred years ago the bowel was thought to be as vital to life as the heart, so removal was seen to spell certain death. Now we know differently – there are many people who have lost part or all of their bowel, yet lead normal, happy and productive lives. However, natural and problem-free function of the bowels is something that most people take for granted and may not appreciate until they have problems. Fortunately there have been great advances in dealing with these problems, both in cancer and non-cancer diseases.

The rectum and anal canal have two main functions: storage and then expulsion of the faeces and flatus.

Storage

This is the main function of the rectum, retaining faeces and flatus until the opportunity comes to empty it. Most people can control the urge, and develop an unconscious timetable to fit **defaecation** into a convenient pattern. For many people this comprises a single morning bowel movement, but there is great individual variation, so there is no such thing as a single 'normal' pattern.

myth
Faeces ('poo') is just the leftovers of digestion.

fact
Up to 80 per cent of it is made up of dead bacteria, which have played a part in digesting food, but which have died and been replaced by others.

defaecation
The process of emptying the rectum via the anus – otherwise delicately known by doctors as 'evacuation' or 'moving the bowel'.

Expulsion of faeces (defaecation) and flatus

It is one of those small miracles of nature that the rectum and anal canal working together can differentiate between wind (flatus) and faeces. Because of this very convenient ability it is possible to pass wind discreetly, often while mingling with other people, and without risking faeces passing out too. When it is appropriate to pass anything, the brain, rectum, anal canal and the abdominal and pelvic muscles work together to engineer (usually) a happy outcome. The process is initiated by a sensation of rectal fullness. Under normal conditions, the urge is suppressed by conscious activity until a decision is taken to 'go'. Then the abdominal muscles (including the diaphragm) may contract; as this occurs, the muscles of the anal canal and the pelvic floor relax automatically to allow passage, after which they resume their normal state of contraction. Passage of flatus is a different matter altogether. Complete, and hopefully fully controlled, sphincter relaxation allows silent passage.

Summary

In essence, then, the large bowel is just a long muscle tube with an absorptive lining. Through evolution, it has developed into a very complex organ that allows us to get rid of the body's gaseous and solid wastes comfortably and in a socially acceptable manner. We have noted that its lining is the tissue most likely to develop cancer. Its nerve supply may give us warnings of disease – cancer or otherwise – while its blood supply and lymphatic drainage play a major part in any spread of cancer.

CHAPTER

2

What is cancer?

One in three people in the Western world will get some form of it in their lifetime and it is now the cause of more than one-quarter of all deaths in Western countries. Cancer is one of the biggest challenges facing modern medicine. Malignant diseases are the second leading cause of all deaths after heart disease. Yet few people would feel confident that they know what cancer is, how best to live their lives to reduce their risk of it, or how to understand and cope with cancer if and when it strikes them, their family or friends.

Listed below are a few useful definitions:

✧ **Tumour** comes from Latin, and simply means a lump. Although it can refer to any lump – due to inflammation, cancer, bony deformity – in modern medical parlance it is mainly used for the sort of 'tumour' we are talking about here, whether malignant or benign.

✧ *Malignant* describes a tumour in which the normal cells are growing so out of control that the resulting lump grows into ('invades') surrounding tissues, within the organ of origin, directly into surrounding organs, or indirectly by escape of malignant cells into the bloodstream so that they reach distant organs.

✧ *Benign* describes a tumour in which the normal cells have started to grow out of control, producing a lump that continues to grow, but does not have the capacity to invade locally or spread elsewhere via the bloodstream.

✧ *Cancer* is derived from the Latin word for crab and is used in a general way for this disease, whichever organ or part of the body is involved.

✧ *Carcinoma* is a more specific term referring only to those cancers arising from the covering and lining tissues of the body ('epithelium') and is derived from the Greek word for crab.

Why this word origin for cancer and carcinoma? There are several possible explanations. The first is that the appearance of the cut surface of a cancerous **mass** may have the appearance of radiating crab's legs; another explanation is the slow leg movements of the crab that conjure up the image of cancer spreading within a person's body.

✧ *Neoplasia* is a word that comes from the Latin meaning 'new growth', and refers to any benign or malignant tumour.

To understand why there are different types of cancer it may be helpful first to consider the make-up of the human body.

myth
All tumours are malignant.

fact
'Tumour' just means 'lump', so many, indeed most, tumours are benign.

myth
Cancer is a death sentence.

fact
True once, but these days some types of cancer are usually cured, while the cure rates for many other types, including bowel, breast and prostate cancer, are improving quite quickly.

mass
Sometimes used instead of 'tumour'.

✧ **Cells** are the basic building blocks of living things and come in many different types. Millions of cells of the same type form:

✧ **Tissues** (for example, muscle, bone, fat, nerve) and several tissue types organized together form:

✧ **Organs**, which are bodily structures made up of several types of tissue that carry out a specific job, for example, heart, lung, brain, bowel.

Cells grow and divide to form new cells as and when needed, under the influence of substances called growth factors and growth inhibitors. So when all is well, tissues and organs are made up of just the right numbers of each type of cell, all working together to perform complex functions. Most cells are actually *programmed* to age and die (a process known as **apoptosis**), just like the whole organism, and are replaced in an orderly fashion; new cells are produced at the rate required to replace the old ones, this rate varying from tissue to tissue.

Cancer is a disease characterized by the abnormal behaviour of cells, in which they grow and multiply in an uncontrolled manner, having escaped the normal process of apoptosis. These cells then tend to spread within and beyond their organ of origin, continuing to ignore the normal regulatory mechanisms. A single cell that becomes 'malignant' has the capacity to multiply and become a malignant mass, which may then destroy normal cells around it, invade into surrounding tissues and organs, and to shed cells into blood vessels and lymphatics that can then travel to other parts of the body (see Figure 2.1).

apoptosis

Otherwise known as 'planned cell death'. An essential bodily process by which normal cells, having performed their set task for a particular length of time (depending on their tissue type), die and are replaced by fresh, efficient new cells.

The cancer at its site of origin is known as the **primary tumour**. When cancer cells travel from the site of origin in the blood or lymphatics secondary tumours may develop in other parts of the body, such as the liver. This process is known as **metastasis**; this word can also be used as an alternative to secondary tumour. This helps us to understand the difference between benign and malignant tumours: a benign tumour is made up of cells growing abnormally, with some loss of control, but it does not infiltrate into surrounding tissues and does not spread ('metastasize').

When we think of a particular cancer we usually think of a specific organ, for example, cancer of the skin or the breast, but it is more correct to think of cancers in terms of the type of tissue from which they arise. For example, the bowel is composed of several types of tissue: epithelium (the inner lining, or 'mucosa'), muscle, nerves, blood vessels, lymph tissue, etc. Although the vast majority of bowel tumours arise from the epithelium, and are therefore classified as carcinomas, there are less common cancers that arise from the other tissues of the bowel. Such cancers may behave quite differently, have different names, and require different approaches to treatment.

As mentioned above, we think that most cancers arise from changes in a single cell. Such cells multiply until thousands and millions constitute a mass that may be noticeable either as a lump or due to its effects on the function of the host organ, or another organ to which it has spread. Most cancers will have been growing for several years before they cause symptoms.

primary tumour
The original malignancy, growing in and around its organ of origin, e.g. the colon or rectum.

metastasis
Process of the spread of cancer cells and the formation of secondary tumours. Also used as another word for a secondary tumour. Often shortened by doctors in conversation to 'met'.

(a)

(b)

(c)

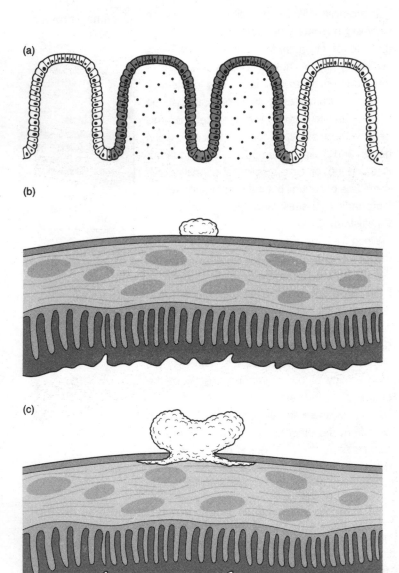

(d)

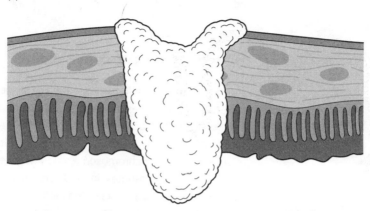

(e)

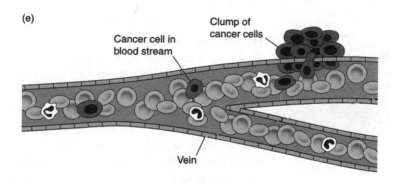

Cancer cell in
blood stream

Clump of
cancer cells

Vein

Figure 2.1 Steps in the development of bowel cancer.
(a) A single bowel lining cell becomes abnormal and
    breeds a small clump of similar cells.
(b) These may grow into a small visible lump
    (adenoma).
(c) This may in turn develop an area of invasive cancer
    within it.
(d) This will enlarge, destroying the adenoma and begin
    to spread into the surrounding tissues.
(e) Cancer cells may enter nearby veins and lymph
    channels to be carried to the liver and beyond.

Sometimes the tumour has metastasized to other parts of the body before any symptoms occur.

mutation
An alteration in the structure of a gene, either inherited or caused during life, that may have an effect on cell function, including triggering malignancy.

cancer family
A family with a high incidence of certain types of cancer, e.g. bowel, due to a genetic mutation.

myth
Cancer always runs in families.

fact
Just because a relative has had cancer, it doesn't mean that you are necessarily more likely to get it. There are so-called 'cancer families' but these give rise to a small proportion of all cancers.

carcinogen
Any substance that can affect the function of cells, leading to their becoming malignant.

How does cancer come about?

A gene is a unit of DNA, the chemical key to the molecular 'memory' responsible for building and maintaining the structure and function of the organism, whether a human or a flea. Thousands of genes make up a chromosome, and there are 23 pairs of chromosomes in each cell in the body, so that every cell contains the full 'blueprint' for the person (or the flea!). In most cancers, changes in one or more of the genes lead to alterations in cell function. These gene changes (**mutations**) may be inherited from parents or they may occur because of damage to genes during a person's lifetime. If a mutation has been inherited, it has been present in every cell in the body since long before birth, and usually leads to cancer at a younger age than usual (30–50 years). Inherited mutations may give rise to cancers in close relatives, and hence to so-called **cancer families**.

In most cancers, however, the mutations are mainly confined to the cells that become the primary tumour, and have been caused by certain substances (**carcinogens**) that have entered our bodies – perhaps in food, smoke, or infections. These may cause very specific damage to particular genes, leading to cells becoming or growing 'out of control', and hence to cancer.

The main suspected environmental factors that either cause, or indirectly expose us to the risk of, cancer include:

✧ personal lifestyle factors (e.g. high fat diets, alcohol, tobacco)

✧ inter-personal factors (e.g. **human papilloma virus**, hepatitis B or C infections)

✧ environmental exposures through work or everyday living (e.g. asbestos, radiation, air pollution).

Often we do not know how carcinogens act, nor do we know the identity of many of the genes they can affect. A gene that can be mutated by a carcinogen to make a cell malignant is called an **oncogene,** and many have been discovered for various types of cancers. There are also genes that decrease any tendency for cells to become malignant – **tumour suppressor genes**.

So what cancer-causing agents have we identified? The best known, of course, is tobacco smoke, the cause of about 90 per cent of lung cancers. Yet we do not know exactly how the inhalation of smoke makes normal cells cancerous. In cancer of the cervix it appears that a virus (the human papilloma virus, HPV) may be an important causative factor. Chewing betel nut is a very common habit in southern and south eastern Asia, leading to large numbers of mouth cancers.

Twenty-five years ago a report called 'The Causes of Cancer' was published by two leading British researchers, Doll and Peto. They believed that cancer death rates could be slashed by attention to known and avoidable causes – certain occupations, infections, and **polluting agents** – but the two most important causes by far were tobacco (30 per cent of all cancer deaths) and diet (35 per cent of all cancer deaths). These

myth
Cancer is avoidable if you avoid all risk factors.

fact
You can certainly improve your chances – just look at smoking – but we don't understand all the causes, so you'll still be at some risk.

human papilloma viruses (HPV)
Group of virus types, some of which cause skin warts while others play a part in the causation of cancer at several sites, principally the cervix, but also the anus and throat.

oncogene
An altered gene that influences other genes to cause cancer.

tumour suppressor gene
Genes with the opposite effect to oncogenes.

polluting agents
Substances released into the environment that can have harmful effects, such as chemical waste, oil, tobacco smoke.

estimates were based largely on indirect evidence from the studies of whole populations of people with and without cancer, looking at differences in the circumstances of the two groups. This kind of research is done by scientists known as epidemiologists, who try to determine the distribution of cancer – who gets it (old/young, male/female, occupation), where (geography), and when (cancer rates vary through history). This sort of information has important lessons for society as it seeks to deal with cancer and health risks.

It is very difficult to prove conclusively the cancer-causing role of 'lifestyle' factors such as the Western diet (high fat, low fibre, low carbohydrate) and identifying these factors is not the same as understanding how cancers come about. Epidemiologists might come up with evidence, for instance, that people who eat a meat-free high-fibre diet are less likely to get bowel cancer, but it is the task of other scientists to work out why. This requires an understanding of what is happening within cells, particularly the parts of the cell that control its growth and replication. This is the work of molecular biologists, geneticists, immunologists, micro-biologists, biochemists, pathologists and many others. We will return to these topics when we discuss some specific theories of the causes of bowel cancer in the next chapter.

Types of cancer

As mentioned earlier, the body is made up of many types of tissue. It is useful to classify cancers according to the kind of tissue from which they arise.

The most common cancers are those that arise from lining and covering tissues (skin, bowel, bladder and lung lining, etc.) – they are collectively called 'carcinomas'. When the lining tissue contains tiny glands that secrete mucus or other substances (epithelium, mucosa), the cancer is called an **adenocarcinoma**. This term covers most tumours arising from the gastrointestinal tract – including the large bowel – the breast, and reproductive systems. Cancers that arise from the supporting structures such as muscle, bone, and connective tissues are classified separately as 'sarcomas'. Thus a malignant tumour arising from bone is called an 'osteosarcoma', and from muscle a 'myosarcoma'. Cancers of the blood and immune system are consigned to other categories ('leukaemias' and 'lymphomas').

> **adenocarcinoma**
> Carcinoma arising from glands (Latin 'adeno' = gland).

What is bowel cancer?

This is a cancer that arises from the internal lining (epithelium, mucosa) of the large bowel (colon and rectum), which is of course in direct contact with the intestinal contents, the faeces, which may be important in the causation of bowel cancer.

Types of bowel cancer

Adenocarcinoma is so much more common than other types of cancer in the bowel that the simpler terms 'bowel cancer' or 'colorectal cancer' are used in everyday medical-speak. Adeno-carcinoma of the large bowel may be divided into two subgroups, cancer of the colon and cancer of the rectum, as there are some

> **myth**
> Cancer is cancer – it's all one disease.

> **fact**
> Just as infectious diseases are different – with different causes, behaviour and seriousness – so it's the same for cancer. There is an enormous number of quite different diseases under the cancer banner.

polyp

A small lump – often on a stalk, like a cherry – growing from an epithelial surface. These can grow in several organs, including the bowel, uterus and nose.

adenoma

Benign tumour arising in glandular lining tissue.

adenomatous polyp

There are several types of polyp that can grow in the bowel, but the adenomatous polyp is the most important because of the link with cancer.

myth

All adenomas become cancers.

fact

Although adenomas are the starting point for almost every bowel cancer, only around one in 20 adenomas turns into a cancer.

dysplasia

Abnormal appearance of cells viewed under the microscope comprising changes in structure typical of benign and malignant tumours.

important differences with respect to diagnosis, treatment and outcome. To the epidemiologist, concerned with understanding the causes and risk factors for bowel cancer, this division is of much less importance. While there is much speculation about differences in the occurrence and causes of cancer of the colon and rectum, their similarities are much more apparent. Therefore, for the purpose of describing their characteristics, we will regard all bowel cancers as constituting the same disease.

More than 90 per cent of bowel cancers arise from glandular epithelium, but there are other types of carcinoma that arise from the lining of the bowel; moreover, tumours rarely arise from other bowel tissues – muscle, fat, blood vessels.

There are several steps in the transition from normal bowel mucosa to an invasive cancer. It is likely that in the earliest stage a single cell multiplies abnormally to form new cells, producing a minute cluster with the same high rate of replication. These cells are not detectable by any test presently available. After a while the abnormal cells form into a small lump (or **polyp**) that constitutes a benign tumour known as an **adenoma** (or **adenomatous polyp**), and these can be single or multiple.

Viewed under a microscope, the cells in an adenoma have certain features that differ from the appearance of normal cells. These differences are referred to as **dysplasia**, which simply means 'abnormal growth'. Most adenomas never grow bigger than a few millimetres and never go on to cause any problem for their host. However, a few adenomas, probably by the accumulation of further genetic changes induced by other factors, grow into larger adenomas. A proportion of large adenomas take a further step into abnormality when cells within them become malignant, leading to the escape of some of those cells from the mucosa into the tissues beneath. The cancerous cells continue to invade, destroying what is left of the benign adenoma, and extending down into the muscle layer of the bowel and beyond. This progression from normal mucosa, through benign and on to malignant transformation, is known as the **adenoma-carcinoma sequence**.

Adenoma-carcinoma sequence

All this raises the question of whether bowel cancer could be prevented by removing adenomas before they can develop into cancer, a very important and controversial question facing health planners and society today. This would be an immense and costly exercise as adenomas are much more common than bowel cancer (one-third of all people over the age of 60 have adenomas in their bowel). Our best guess is that less than five per cent of all adenomas develop into cancer, and that the time from the origin of an adenoma until the development of cancer may be between five and ten years. So, what should these facts mean in terms of practical policy? As it is technically feasible to find such adenomas and remove them quite safely, should we implement a programme of aggressive detection and removal of adenomas to try to prevent bowel cancer altogether? This question will be discussed in the chapter on screening and prevention.

adenoma-carcinoma sequence (ACS)
Process by which normal tissue enters the pathway to cancer, starting as a benign tumour (adenoma), which grows and then becomes malignant (carcinoma). The ACS is driven by an accumulation of gene mutations.

How does bowel cancer progress?

Q Don't all cancers progress at the same rate?

A No. Some types grow and spread much faster than others, and even with individual cancer types, including bowel cancer, there are some tumours that are much more 'aggressive' than others.

average survival
Individual patients survive for different periods – if you add all the individual lengths of survival and divide by the number of patients you get the 'average' length of survival. This is something used by doctors to discuss prospects for patients, while highlighting the variability there is in survival.

invasion
In this context we are referring to the tendency for malignant cancer cells to spread into neighbouring tissues and organs.

fistula
An abnormal opening between two organs or surfaces, through which bodily fluids can leak. Examples include 'colovesical' (colon to bladder), 'rectovaginal' (rectum to vagina), 'enterocutaneous' (bowel, small or large, to skin).

Almost no patient is beyond any treatment for this disease today, but in decades and centuries gone by, this was not the case. In 1964, a study was published that looked at the fate of patients in history who had not undergone surgical treatment. Interestingly, symptoms had been present for an average of eight months prior to diagnosis, much as is the case today. However, the prospects for patients were dramatically different back then: the **average survival** after diagnosis was just ten months, with less than 25 per cent surviving for a year, and only two per cent for five years. Today more than 50 per cent of those undergoing treatment are cured.

Broadly we divide the progression of bowel cancer into two phases – local and distant spread – though in some patients these phases can occur simultaneously.

Local spread

As the tumour grows, it spreads out through the bowel wall to **invade** surrounding tissues. In some cases the tumour can invade nearby organs. This invasive process is naturally known as local spread. In men with rectal cancer, the bladder and prostate may thus be invaded. Occasionally a rectal cancer will extend to the inner lining of the bladder, causing bleeding or infection in the urine, or even leakage of faeces and gas into the bladder (i.e. a **fistula** has developed), which will be passed in the urine. In women the vagina and uterus lie between the rectum and bladder, thus protecting the latter. Invasion of the vagina may lead to a fistula, and leakage of faeces into (and out of) the vagina.

Thankfully all these complications are quite uncommon. Local spread of rectal cancer may also affect the small bowel (as it lies in the lower abdominal cavity against the front wall of the rectum), and the side walls of the pelvis where the muscles, nerves, and bones may be invaded.

Colon cancer may invade the various structures lying behind it on the back wall of the abdominal cavity, including the ureters and the duodenum. Again, the small bowel, which lies in close contact with the colon, may be invaded.

Distant spread

The organ most commonly involved in distant spread via the bloodstream is the liver, which is found to harbour secondary tumours (metastases) in around 30 per cent of patients at the time of initial diagnosis. A further 30 per cent of patients are likely to develop liver metastases at some time after primary treatment due to growth from microscopic and undetectable deposits of cancer cells that were already present in the liver at the time of initial diagnosis. Liver metastases may be curable surgically though not if they are widespread; advances in liver surgery mean that 30 per cent of patients operated on are cured.

Another important site for spread from bowel cancer is the peritoneal membrane lining the abdominal cavity, resulting from cells shed from the surface of the tumour after it has invaded through the full thickness of the bowel wall. **Peritoneal deposits** sometimes cause the production of fluid in the abdominal cavity (**ascites**) which may cause marked distension of the abdomen.

The next most common site for distant spread is the lungs, though these are involved in only

Q **Don't all cancers spread distantly eventually?**

A No. Some cancer types just spread locally and if left untreated would never spread. This rule applies, for instance, to one sort of skin cancer. In other cases, including bowel cancer, we can't tell in individual patients, so that frequently we give drugs to kill any hidden cells around the body just to make sure.

peritoneal deposits
Nodules of tumour growing on the inner lining of the abdomen.

ascites
Collection of fluid in the abdominal cavity. Can be due to cancer, liver disease and occasionally heart failure.

about ten per cent of patients, mostly at a late stage in the disease. If near the surface of the lung, secondary tumours may cause a collection of fluid within the chest cavity, compressing the lung and causing shortness of breath.

Bowel cancer can spread to any other part of the body via the bloodstream, though this occurs much less frequently than with cancers of the breast and lung.

Summary

In this chapter we have examined the nature of cancer, in general and in the bowel, how it comes about, and something of its patterns of behaviour in the body. We have had a cursory glance at the causes and mechanisms; next we will go into these aspects in more detail.

CHAPTER

3

What are the causes of bowel cancer?

Modern treatment saves many lives, and the chances of surviving bowel cancer are slowly getting better. Prevention is always preferable to cure, but prevention is facilitated by an understanding of the causes and mechanisms of a disease. In the nineteenth century there were some weird and wonderful ideas about the causes of life-threatening infections, but it was only when they came to understand the existence and behaviour of 'germs' that the conquest of many infectious diseases became possible. The same will be true for cancer – when we know just how bowel cancer comes about, then we should be able to combat the disease at its source.

We have known for a long time that there are things about the way we live that play a part in bowel cancer. We have also known for a long time that our genetic make-up may play a part, especially in those rare families in which bowel cancer afflicts up to half their members. We are also coming to understand that in many more people there are more subtle features of our genes that can interact with environmental, especially dietary, factors, making it more – or less – likely that we will be affected.

A world view of bowel cancer

There are many clues to be uncovered simply by comparing the way the disease affects people in different parts of the world. Globally there are around one million new cases of bowel cancer each year and half a million deaths. Yet it is rare amongst the majority of the world's people, particularly in Africa and Asia. It is most common in western Europe, North America, Australasia and South Africa. In the UK there are currently about 34,000 new cases of bowel cancer and 17,000 deaths each year; here it accounts for about ten per cent of all cancer deaths and is second only to lung cancer. Around one in 20 Britons will develop bowel cancer, and one in 50 will die of it. However, looking at the rest of the world, globally there are still four cases of tuberculosis for every case of bowel cancer, while in the West there are about 10 bowel cancer cases for every case of TB. In rural Africa ten people die in road accidents for every one bowel cancer death. All this suggests strongly that there is something about the Western way of life that puts the population at excess risk for bowel cancer.

More evidence comes from those populations that have migrated from low to high risk countries such as the African slaves and their descendants who now live in the US, and the Japanese who moved to Hawaii and the US West Coast in the early to mid twentieth century. These people took on the risk level of their adopted countries, strongly suggesting that it was their new environment, probably including their diet, that generated the risk. If yet more evidence is wanted, we should note the increasing prevalence of the disease in countries, or parts of countries, that are 'westernizing'. In Japan the disease increased threefold between 1960 and 1980 – in one generation Japan has gone from being a low risk country to one of those with the highest risk; and in China bowel cancer is also increasing.

It is not just in bowel cancer that environmental factors play a big part: they are important in several cancer types, and may be found in people's circumstances, habits and lifestyle. For a start, there are those factors similarly affecting large swathes of the world, such as climate, but although we know sunlight has a major causative effect in skin cancer, it cannot be a factor in bowel cancer – otherwise it would be as common in Calcutta as Canberra. No, bowel cancer appears to be much more 'personal' than that; within low risk countries it is more common amongst the rich and urbanized than in their poverty stricken countrymen. So what is it about the 'individual environment'? What about personal circumstances such as hygiene and sexual activity? We know that cervical cancer is much more common in sexually active women than in nuns – this is wholly down to the sexually transmitted human papilloma virus (HPV). What about smoking? Certainly for lung cancer, much less in bowel cancer.

So just what is it in bowel cancer? By far the most likely factors appear to relate to diet – what we eat and how we digest it. After all, the bowel lining, where cancer develops, has our food, the digestive juices, and the products of digestion as its most intimate neighbours. For many years now, the elements of the highly **refined diet** born of industrialized agriculture and food processing have been the number one suspects in the hunt for the causes of bowel cancer.

If the Western diet is the main culprit it would be expected that the disease became more common in Western countries as this diet evolved – and, though data are sparse, this appears to be so. So we need to explore our diet looking for more clues.

What is it about what we eat?

Evidence has been building up slowly for a long time, but much of it is circumstantial rather than based on precise scientific fact, so it is difficult to give firm dietary advice on what would decrease the risk of bowel cancer. Also, to complicate matters, it is becoming clear that in some people their genes, especially those that control the body's digestion and **metabolism**, play a big part in whether or not we are individually more susceptible to these dietary factors. So what has come to light through years of effort to define dietary risk?

Dietary elements that may increase the risk of bowel cancer

Cancer promoters and cancer initiators

We know there are substances in our food that may start the cancer process (the **initiators**) while others drive the process once it has started

refined diet
Range of foodstuffs produced by industrialized food industry, and including many foods in which 'refining' has removed constituents including fibre (e.g. most white bread flours).

metabolism
Bodily processes that break down food materials into useable substances (glucose, amino acids, etc) and neutralize and excrete potentially harmful waste products.

initiator
Substance that can start the process of cell change leading to cancer.

(the **promoters**). There are certainly low concentrations of initiators ('carcinogens') in our environment; for instance, the charring of red meat on the grill or barbecue may cause the production of one or more carcinogens. Precisely how major dietary elements have their effect is unclear, but some of the suspects are high dietary fat, red meat and alcohol.

promoter
Substance that drives forward cellular changes towards cancer after it has been started by an initiator.

High dietary fat

In countries with a high incidence of bowel cancer, large amounts of meat and animal fat are consumed. This is, of course, not sufficient evidence to prove a cause and effect since there are other factors common to these countries that might be responsible (after all, television sets are also much more common in 'bowel cancer countries', but no one has yet come up with this as a cause of the disease!). Several studies have looked at animal fat and have shown a relationship between total fat consumption and bowel cancer risk, though chemical type of fat or calorie load might play a part. It is likely that the effect of fat is not direct (fat itself does not cause cancers to appear or grow) but indirect, by its stimulation of bile production by the liver. It is also well established that obesity is associated with an increased risk of bowel cancer.

Fatty acids are some of the building blocks of fat molecules. For a long time it has been thought that saturated fatty acids may play a part in bowel cancer risk, and that we are best advised to consume fats containing unsaturated fatty acids (one in particular is called omega 3). Nevertheless, in a very large analysis published in 2006, looking at nearly 50,000 people

fatty acids
Long molecules that form the building blocks of natural dietary fats and oils.

considered in many smaller studies, it would appear the basis for this advice is far from proven.

What are bile acids and what is their role in bowel cancer?

The bowel lining is covered in the bacteria that aid digestion, and is bathed in the chemicals that digest our food – these include the **bile acids**, present in the **bile** produced by the liver, and it appears that they may play a part in the development of bowel cancer. They aid fat digestion by breaking it up into minute globules ('emulsification'), which are easier to digest and absorb. The presence of fat in the intestine encourages the liver to produce more bile acids to promote its digestion. Certain bacteria in the bowel are able to convert the bile acids and cholesterol into a form that can actively promote the growth of existing small adenomas into larger ones, which are more likely to develop into cancers.

bile acids
Substances in bile that aid digestion of fat by breaking it up into very fine globules, giving a much larger surface area for reaction with fat digesting chemicals ('enzymes').

bile
Green or brown fluid produced by the liver, and delivered into the upper intestinal tract. Contains bile acids and several waste products (bilirubin and cholesterol) for voiding in the faeces.

Red meat

This has been on the suspect list for many years. Why red meat rather than other protein sources – such as fish or white meat? It may well be related to its particular fat content, or it could be due to the chemicals produced during cooking, particularly if the meat is charred. More recently, processed meats – ham, bacon, luncheon meats – have come under suspicion.

Alcohol

Heavy drinking over prolonged periods has been associated with increased risk, perhaps by as much as 25 per cent.

What may decrease the risk of bowel cancer?

Dietary fibre

This has been top of the healthy list for many decades, though the circumstantial evidence for it has been somewhat dented by more recent studies. **Dietary fibre** is a broadly used term for substances of plant origin that are not digested, so they end up forming a large proportion of our faeces. Our usual sources include the bran of wheat (from the husk of the seed) and the fibrous parts of some fruits and vegetables. You might think it unlikely that a food substance that is not metabolized or absorbed into our bodies could be important to our health! Yet many believe that increasing the fibre content of our diet is one of the most important preventive measures we can take, not only against bowel cancer but many other diseases as well.

> **dietary fibre**
> Indigestable food element, principally found in cereals and certain fruit and vegetables, that add bulk to, and soften, the stool. Lost in process of food refining.

In the 1970s Denis Burkitt, an English surgeon who was working in Africa, produced some of the main evidence; one aspect of his work involved collecting and characterizing human stools deposited in the African bush, and comparing them with the stools of pupils in British public schools. He found the former to be bulkier, faster in transit and less odorous. He put all this down to differences in fibre intake, bolstering the 'fibre is good for you' hypothesis, and suggesting a preventive role in bowel cancer.

The debate has been lucrative for those who produce and distribute fibre-rich foods, but its value for the people consuming bran and the like has yet to be proven fully. For the moment, if you are someone who opts for things that may make you more healthy or may protect you, you

EPIC study

Enormous European study tracking the health of 500,000 healthy volunteers to ascertain factors associated with cancer risk, including dietary elements, alcohol, smoking, exercise, medications, etc. Has produced supportive data for many of the assertions in this chapter.

myth

Eat enough fruit and vegetables and you won't get bowel cancer.

fact

This might decrease the risk, but it is not completely protective. Much of the evidence about fruit and vegetables is circumstantial.

cruciferous vegetables

Include broccoli, Brussels sprouts and cauliflower that are high in natural fibre.

chemoprotective agent

Substance that may decrease the risk of cancer development.

will be one of the millions who go for high-fibre foods.

There is a major study involving over 500,000 people going on in the UK and eight other European countries. It is looking at the relationship between diet, lifestyle and cancer. This study is called **EPIC** (The European Prospective Investigation of Cancer). It started in 1992 and will produce reports on how diet and lifestyle relate to a variety of cancers over a period of decades, starting with bowel cancer and breast cancer.

Fruit and vegetables

Of course, people who eat less meat tend to eat more vegetables, and it is possible that any reduction in risk for bowel cancer among non-meat eaters is due to a protective effect of vegetables, and this may be due to more than their fibre content. Some animal research has shown that the addition of **cruciferous vegetables** (broccoli, Brussels sprouts, cauliflower) can protect against certain cancers. Some studies in humans have shown that the risk of bowel cancer can be reduced by as much as 25 per cent in people who eat large amounts of vegetables. Some of the vegetable effect is likely to be due to the fibre found in many types, but a **chemoprotective** effect may occur due to the presence of certain other substances. It is usual advice to eat at least five portions of fruit and/or vegetables daily.

Vitamins and trace elements

There is evidence that certain vitamins and so-called 'trace elements' – substances present in the body in minute amounts that play a crucial part in the workings of the body – may help to prevent or slow the growth of tumours. Vitamin A (retinol), Vitamin C, calcium and selenium have all been cited. At present, the data suggesting **chemopreventive** roles for these substances have come mainly from studies of tumours in animals, though there are studies under way to look at their role in humans, particularly in the prevention or inhibition of growth of adenomas. Calcium may protect against bowel cancer; a research review in 2004 found that including about one gram of calcium in your diet every day might help to decrease the formation of adenomas and hence reduce bowel cancer incidence.

Summary – diet and bowel cancer

There are lots of unanswered questions in this complex scientific story. However, the most likely series of events leading to bowel cancer includes the initiation of small adenomas due to genetic factors by environmental carcinogens, and the growth of some of these in appropriate conditions to form large adenomas, and then cancer. These stages are likely to be encouraged by dietary fat, which increases the amount of bile acids and cholesterol in the bowel. These substances are probably acted upon by bacteria to produce cancer promoters. Some food constituents, particularly fibre, may diminish the effects of the promoters, in the case of fibre by hurrying them out of the bowel. Interestingly, low-fat, high fibre, and fruit and vegetable rich diets are also associated with lower rates of coronary artery disease and other diseases.

myth

Take enough vitamins from the health food shop and you'll be protected from all sorts of diseases, including bowel cancer.

fact

This will prevent so-called vitamin deficiency diseases, but its role in cancer prevention remains very much open to question.

chemopreventive agent

Substance with capacity to prevent cancer development (i.e. one step on from chemoprotection).

Non-steroidal anti-inflammatory drugs (NSAIDs)

These widely used medicines relieve pain in arthritis, headaches, back strain and menstruation. Aspirin, the best known, is also used to thin the blood to decrease the risk of heart attacks and strokes. Certain varieties of NSAIDs have been suggested to protect against bowel cancer through their suppression of adenoma development. These drugs ('COX-2 inhibitors') are thought to inhibit the action of an enzyme called COX-2. There are studies going on throughout the world to see if taking these drugs will prevent more polyps forming in people who have already had them removed.

One trial called CAPP 2 is testing aspirin and corn starch in people who carry the HNPCC gene (see page 44) and who therefore have a high risk of bowel cancer. This trial finished recruiting in June 2005, but it will be some time before we know the results. Another trial called VICTOR was looking at giving an anti-inflammatory drug called rofecoxib to try to stop bowel cancer coming back after surgery. Unfortunately this trial had to be stopped early because the researchers observed increased side effects and the pharmaceutical company withdrew the drug. The role of NSAIDs in chemoprevention of bowel cancer is still unresolved.

Genes and bowel cancer

We have known for a long time that diet and the environment are not the whole story: in particular, we have known for decades that our genetic make-up may predispose us to bowel cancer. In the past 25 years this has become a very important area of laboratory research, and has

Q **I've been told I'm a member of a bowel cancer family. Does that mean my children and I are bound to get bowel cancer?**

A Around half of the offspring of cancer patients in cancer families will develop the disease unless preventive measures are taken. If you haven't inherited the defective gene (and sometimes tests can show whether you have or not), you can't pass it on to your children – your line has lost the risk. However, you can still get bowel cancer due to environmental factors, just like anyone else in the population.

given us wider insight into the molecular mechanisms underlying not just family cancers but the generality of cases.

Early in the twentieth century a condition known now as **familial adenomatous polyposis (FAP)** was recognized, in which bowel cancer developed by the age of 40 in affected people, and in which half the children of such people could be expected to inherit the condition (**dominant inheritance**). Around one in 10,000 people are born with FAP, in which the colon and rectum become carpeted in thousands of adenomas, usually by the age of 15, and it is only a matter of time before one or more of these becomes cancerous if the condition is not recognized and treated. In the early days this disease was untreatable, but in the 1940s surgeons began to remove much of the affected bowel before the onset of cancer, thus greatly decreasing the risk that cancer would ever develop. It was understood decades ago that FAP was due to just one defective gene out of the 50,000 we carry in each cell in our bodies. In the late 1980s the gene was identified; later it was found that the normally functioning gene is a 'tumour suppressor' – in other words it acts to minimize the tendency for abnormal, potentially malignant, cell behaviour to occur. So if the gene is not working properly, that protective effect is lost. Today it is possible to perform laboratory tests in family members in order to make the diagnosis before the adenomas have developed. Previously the shadow of the disease hung over all those at risk, whereas by using a blood test we can now at least set the minds at rest of the 50 per cent of family members *not* carrying the gene defect.

familial adenomatous polyposis (FAP)
Rare inherited condition, characterized by the development of thousands of adenomas in the large bowel, and to a lesser extent in the duodenum. Progression to bowel cancer by the age of 40 is certain if not diagnosed and treated.

dominant inheritance
Pattern of inheritance in which there is a 50 per cent chance that each child of an affected person will inherit the condition.

hereditary non-polyposis colorectal cancer syndrome (HNPCC)

Another dominantly inherited condition causing bowel cancer.

Q **Why should cancer develop earlier than average in cancer family members?**

A The average age for onset of bowel cancer is 70 years. It takes this time to get enough genetic damage from the environment to develop cancer. Unfortunately, in cancer families they have a 'head start', having inherited key causative defective genes, so it takes less time to collect the whole set.

FAP is easily diagnosed – no other condition produces such a mass of adenomas in the large bowel. A more insidious condition has been recognized that also carries a 50 per cent risk of inheritance in affected families, but which does not lead to the thousands of adenomas seen in FAP. Indeed, in an affected individual the disease looks like any other case of bowel cancer in the general population. The condition carries the snappy name of **hereditary non-polyposis colorectal cancer syndrome (HNPCC)**. The giveaways are that the cancer usually appears by the age of 30 to 50, and the patient is likely to have close relatives who have, or have had, bowel cancer, or cancer of the uterus, ovary, pancreas, urinary tract or stomach. There are formal criteria that help to decide whether a particular family is affected by HNPCC: they are known as the 'modified Amsterdam' or 'Bethesda' criteria, named after places where expert groups produced them. The criteria are:

◇ at least two generations having cancer cases
◇ three or more relatives affected
◇ at least one individual affected before the age of 50
◇ at least one individual had bowel cancer, though the rest could have harboured the associated cancers.

As a routine, doctors coming across young people (certainly up to the age of 45) with bowel cancer, or those with two or more close relatives with bowel cancer or the associated tumours mentioned above, should be alert to the risk to other family members and arrange for them to be examined.

The genetic basis for HNPCC has also been identified. Amazingly, every time a new cell is made, its newly constructed gene pool is checked for mistakes in production; any mistake is literally chopped out and a correct piece of DNA is put in its place (**mismatch repair**, MMR). This process is occurring millions of times a second as new cells are made. It has been found that a breakdown in this seek-and-repair mechanism occurs in HNPCC due to an inherited mutation on one of several genes, known as MLH1, MSH2, MSH6. As a result of failure of MMR, genetic mistakes – mutations – survive unrepaired, leading ultimately to abnormal cell growth and, in some cases, to the birth of cancer cells. Members of some HNPCC families can be identified and offered regular bowel examination by colonoscopy; removal of adenomas means that these benign tumours cannot go on to become malignant. So long as this examination is repeated three yearly, cancer can be very effectively prevented. If cancer does develop, requiring surgery, there is the option to remove much of the colon, as in FAP, thereby permanently decreasing the risk of future cancers.

mismatch repair
Extraordinary example of the complexity of cell biology. Process by which mistakes in DNA manufacture are detected and repaired. Loss of this mechanism forms the basis of cancer predisposition on HNPCC.

While FAP and HNPCC account for around five per cent of all bowel cancers, there are certainly more cases – perhaps another 20 per cent of them – in which less 'powerful', and often multiple, gene mutations conspire to produce cancers in affected families. Usually the pattern of inheritance is not as obvious as in FAP and HNPCC; families of anyone developing bowel cancer below the age of 45, or where two or more close relatives develop the disease are best advised to seek medical assessment, probably leading to regular colonoscopy, as occurs in HNPCC families.

What else might affect the risk of getting bowel cancer?

Social and economic factors

Whereas many diseases that afflict humankind are a bigger problem for the poor than the rich, bowel cancer is in some ways an exception. On an international basis, it is clearly a disease of the developed, industrialized countries that enjoy a higher average standard of living. Although socio-economic status within countries does not appear to have a major effect on bowel cancer incidence, there is good evidence that a degree of affluence affects prospects of survival, perhaps related to access to medical services or other factors.

Inflammatory bowel diseases (IBD)

inflammatory bowel disease (IBD)
Persistent inflammatory conditions affecting the intestine, and of ill understood origin, such as ulcerative colitis (UC) and Crohn's disease, present an increased cancer risk for patients.

Patients with long-standing, extensive **inflammatory bowel disease** are known to have an increased risk of getting bowel cancer, although the reasons for this are not clear.

Ulcerative colitis (UC)

Ulcerative colitis is a chronic disease of the large bowel in which the inner lining becomes inflamed and ulcerated. This results in recurring symptoms of diarrhoea and bleeding. Patients with long-standing severe UC are at increased risk of developing cancer – about ten times that of people with 'normal' bowels.

Crohn's disease

Crohn's disease of the colon is the other important chronic inflammatory disease of the large bowel. Crohn's disease can affect any part of the gastrointestinal tract (most commonly the small bowel) and is associated with an increased risk of cancer of the large bowel (probably about twice that of the 'normal' population).

Exercise

Studies have linked physical exercise to a lower risk of colon cancer, but not rectal cancer. Results from the EPIC study so far continue to show there is strong evidence that exercise is associated with a decreased risk of bowel cancer and breast cancer.

Statins

Statins are drugs that are used to lower the level of cholesterol in the blood. Cholesterol is a chemical that is made in the liver from fatty foods. Because statins can lower blood cholesterol, they are used to try to prevent heart disease and strokes. Some researchers have shown that they may have a role in preventing bowel cancer, while other studies suggest either a slight increase or no reduction in cancer for people taking statins. The jury is still out.

So who does get bowel cancer?

Common thoughts in cancer patients and their relatives are: 'Why me?', or, 'Why us?' 'What have I done to deserve this?' Sometimes the 'off-the-cuff' medical answer is: 'Well, it's just one of those

Q Most people eat roughly the same diet in any one country. So why do some get bowel cancer and not others?

A Good question. We think it is because some people's systems get rid of cancer-causing substances more efficiently than others, and this is almost certainly due to inheritance or not of a whole range of genes that play a part in these processes; inherit enough of the relevant genes and you are at much higher risk. In short, some people may just be dealt a bad hand, and start out with a higher risk than others.

things,' or 'It's not your fault', or 'We don't know, but the important thing now is to get on with treatment so that we can get you back to health.'

With more thought it is usually possible to give more helpful answers than these. With all the foregoing evidence in mind, let us look at the whole population and try to pick out any groups known to be at particular risk of bowel cancer.

What effect does our age have on bowel cancer risk?

Despite decades of effort to work out factors that put an individual at increased risk of bowel cancer, and despite all the evidence discussed earlier indicating that some populations are at greater risk than others, when it comes down to individual risk the most important predictor remains a rather simple one – a person's age. The older we get, the higher our chances of getting bowel cancer. It is very rare before the age of 40: less than three per cent of all cases in the UK occur below that age. The average age at diagnosis is about 70 years. The rate of occurrence rises consistently with age; its rate of increase is similar to that of other cancers of the lining tissues of the body that are exposed to cancer-causing agents (for example, smoke and lung cancer, ultraviolet light and skin cancer). This pattern is consistent with theories of dietary or faecal cancer-causing substances that the bowel is repeatedly exposed to, but which take a relatively long time to exert any effect. A corollary of this theory is that cases occurring before the fifth decade of life (40s) are less likely to be due primarily to dietary/environmental factors, and therefore that genetic influences may be relatively more important in this age group.

What about gender?

Although both sexes are at very similar risk for large bowel cancer, there are differences that may prove important in our understanding of the disease. In most countries, rectal cancer is slightly more common in men, whereas colon cancer is slightly more common in women. These differences, however, are affected by age. Beyond the age of 65, there are more cases of both colon and rectal cancer in women. This is because women on average live longer than men in most countries (i.e. there are more old women than old men). When the incidence rate is considered (to cancel out the effect of there being more older women), both colon and rectal cancer are more common in men than women after the age of 65. One explanation for this might be that men, for some reason, become progressively more exposed to the cancer-causing agent(s) than women in later years. At the moment there is no hard evidence in this area.

How important is a family history of bowel cancer?

We discussed this earlier, but it is easy to get it out of proportion. We should emphasize that, although a history of bowel cancer in the family is relevant for some patients, the great majority of cases appear to be **sporadic**, that is, they are not the result of an apparent inherited cause or pattern. Bowel cancer is sufficiently common that many people will have a relative that has had this disease. Having one relative who has had the disease around the average age (70), certainly does not indicate any significant extra risk.

sporadic
In this context it refers to cancers not thought to have an hereditary basis, i.e. occurring randomly, for no obvious genetic reason.

What about social, occupational and economic factors?

As discussed earlier, these factors are important. An illustration of their likely effect within one country, Finland, is a clear example. In Finland, a country with a relatively high incidence of bowel cancer, farmers have only 60 per cent of the average rate of colon cancers, whereas managerial employees have about 25 per cent more than average; self-employed persons (other than farmers) have 67 per cent more bowel cancers. Amongst those who get bowel cancer, wealth appears to be an advantage; studies carried out in the UK have shown that the more affluent are more likely to survive their cancers, probably related to success in gaining access to quality care, but other factors may apply.

Summary

Bowel cancer is predominantly a disease of industrialized Western countries, though it is beginning to make an appearance in the developing countries of the world. There is much circumstantial evidence to suggest that this pattern is related to the lifestyle of the affluent countries and, in particular, the refined diet that has resulted from industrialization of food production. Genetic predisposition and the role of predisposing inflammatory diseases are areas of importance as an understanding of their mechanisms of action may help us to understand the disease process more clearly, while recognition of those at risk due to various factors may allow us to prevent cancer in these people.

CHAPTER

4

Prevention and screening in bowel cancer

'An ounce of prevention is worth a pound of cure' is the sort of saying which seems to ooze good sense, so it should never be a surprise to hear that prevention is to play a much greater part in health care in the future. However, for the moment, success in changing the lifestyles of whole populations has been limited, although tobacco reduction has been successful in many circumstances. Treatment of bowel cancer, once it has reached the stage at which symptoms develop, is successful in only some patients, so efforts to prevent the disease or to detect it earlier by screening have been intensively researched in the last 20 years.

The terms 'prevention' and 'screening' are sometimes used rather loosely.

✧ **Primary prevention** of bowel cancer refers to attempts to block the whole train of events from the earliest cellular changes in

primary prevention
Prevention of cancer by preventing the benign precursor (in this case, the adenoma).

order to prevent triggering of the adenoma cancer sequence.

secondary prevention (screening)

The process of applying a test to a population of symptom-free people to diagnose tumours early to allow more effective treatment.

◇ **Secondary prevention (screening)** has the same important practical outcome, the prevention of advanced cancer, but involves detecting and removing benign adenomas to prevent them developing into cancer, or to identify cancers at a less advanced stage when the chance of cure is higher. The aim is not to prevent the tumour but rather to prevent death from cancer by early diagnosis and more effective treatment. The screening process is applied to symptom-free people, and ideally performed widely as a public health and primary care programme.

Secondary prevention and screening sometimes overlap as we will see shortly.

Primary prevention

Primary prevention works best if we know one or more ways to prevent a disease from occuring. Knowing that pasteurizing milk kills the germ causing tuberculosis is a classical form of primary prevention, as is childhood immunization. Even though we don't know exactly how cigarette smoke induces lung cancer, we can aim at primary prevention by encouraging people not to smoke.

Let's look at primary prevention as it might be applied to bowel cancer. The first major problem is our relative lack of knowledge of how the disease develops at a cellular level. We know that cancer develops through changes in the genes inside our cells, altering the rate of cell growth and multiplication. If we are to understand in order to prevent, therefore, we have to know which genes are affected and how. 'Which genes' is a question that has begun to yield answers. Some very important offender genes that are subject to inherited abnormalities have been identified in the past 20 years, such as those described in Chapter 3, but there are others to find. For the moment, however, the nearest we can get to primary prevention in the cancer-causing genetic conditions is to try to identify involved families and to offer **genetic counselling** to those at risk, and to apply secondary prevention before symptoms occur by removing adenomas either via the colonoscope or by surgical resection. In the future it may become possible to offer some specific 'antidotes' to the effects of such genes.

Another important aspect of primary prevention in bowel cancer relates to the action of agents that may cause gene damage in those born with 'normal' genes. There is much evidence and speculation on the role of a series of dietary factors in this regard. People's dietary habits, evolved and ingrained through their lifetimes, are difficult to record for research purposes and difficult to change for possible cancer prevention. It is likely that in order to produce a sufficient change in diet to diminish bowel cancer risk, we would have to 'eat African' (low fat, high fibre diet) – in other words, take on the whole dietary approach of a low-bowel cancer incidence area. Studies are in progress in large populations to look at the effects of dietary additives such as calcium salts. In addition to the likelihood of reduced incidence of bowel cancer, a 'healthy diet' should also reduce the rates of diabetes, obesity, heart disease, stroke and osteoarthritis.

> **genetic counselling**
> A process of careful collection of family cancer history to plot a detailed family tree, so that detailed and understandable advice can be given to an individual and their family regarding their cancer risks and how to deal with them.

Secondary prevention or screening

Over the past 30 years an enormous research effort has been applied to secondary prevention and screening to see whether early detection and treatment of adenomas and less advanced cancers in symptomless people decreases the death rate from bowel cancer in whole populations.

There is good evidence, particularly from Iceland and the Nordic countries (Sweden, Norway, Denmark and Finland), that the death rate from cervical cancer can be cut dramatically through national screening programmes. Iceland has played a leading role in the implementation of cervical cancer screening – it and the other Nordic countries are particularly efficient in this regard, and have reaped the reward accordingly. In the mid-1980s a national breast cancer screening programme was implemented in the UK, and this played a major role in the decreased death rate for this disease over the past 20 years.

Large clinical trials across the world have shown that the death rate from bowel cancer can be cut by 15 to 20 per cent by the systematic application of one method of bowel cancer screening; this led to pilot studies in the UK to demonstrate that screening can be handled in the NHS. The NHS Bowel Cancer Screening Programme launched in 2006, and is scheduled to be fully operational by 2008. Major improvements in infrastructure have been, and still are, required to support this nationwide.

General issues in screening

Before a government, health service, medical community or general population should accept that

myth

If I get screened and it's negative, it means I haven't got cancer and never will have.

fact

A negative screening test is certainly good news, but like all medical tests, screening is not perfect, and some cancers can be missed. Also, with the FOBt (see opposite), you are no less likely to develop cancer in the future than those not screened. So remain vigilant: watch out for possible symptoms, and see a doctor if they occur.

a mass screening programme (for any condition) should be set up, inviting everyone in the population of the appropriate sex and age to be tested, it is important to establish that the potential benefits of such a programme would outweigh potential harm, and also that it would be a good use of health resources. This can be very difficult to prove, largely because the objective measurement of benefits and harms of medical interventions always requires large and complex research studies. The politicians and administrators of the NHS tread very warily even when the research evidence supports national implementation, ever mindful of the high profile 'failures' that have previously occurred in the delivery of national breast and cervical cancer screening. Such programmes demand the highest quality in all aspects, not only to offer the best chance of detection and early treatment to those with cancer but also, importantly, to avoid harm to those having the tests who turn out *not* to have the target condition.

Faecal occult blood test (FOBt)

So far the main thrust has been to try to identify cancers at the earliest stage, when they are not causing any symptoms. This has centred around a chemical test to detect hidden blood in the bowel motion, the so-called **faecal occult blood test (FOBt)**; this exploits the fact that most bowel cancers bleed slightly, so slightly that it cannot be seen by the naked eye. The test involves applying chemicals to a sample of stool: if a blue coloration appears around the stool specimen the test is positive. This occurs in about one in every 50 tests. A positive does *not* automatically mean that the person harbours a bowel cancer – far from it.

> **faecal occult blood test (FOBt)**
> A simple test to detect invisibly small amounts of blood in faeces as a sign of possible cancer.

However, it *does* mean that they are at a much higher risk than someone whose test was negative; one in ten positive tests is due to a cancer, the rest resulting from piles, traces of animal blood from food, chemicals derived from certain vegetables that can falsely trigger the test, and a few other things as well. So, in those who have tested positive, the hunt is then on for that one in ten. This usually requires them all to undergo a **colonoscopy** to examine the bowel lining in detail.

When the programme is fully implemented, all UK citizens in the 60–69 age range will be sent a test kit (see Figure 4.1) and this will be repeated two yearly. Others are developing similar programmes. In Canada, for instance, the Province of Manitoba has announced its intention to screen persons aged 50–74. The **screenee** will be asked to obtain two pea-sized samples of stool, using a small disposable spatula; this is best achieved by placing newspaper in the lavatory bowl to prevent a stool from diving immediately to the depths. The samples are then placed on the first card. This procedure is repeated on three consecutive days; the cards fold very conveniently to seal away the samples, and are then returned together by post to the laboratory. Each card comes impregnated

colonoscopy
A thorough examination of the inside of the colon and rectum using a long flexible 'telescope', which allows not only an excellent view but also the ability to take samples ('biopsies').

screenee
The person who is the subject of the screening test.

my experience

When I was sent a screening test through the post, there was no way I was going to mess around in the toilet collecting poo, and I told my doctor that when I went to see her about my arthritis. She told me that bowel cancer is very common, and that this test should save 10 to 15 people from dying of bowel cancer *every day* in this country. That was enough for me; so I went home and did it, even though I didn't like the idea.

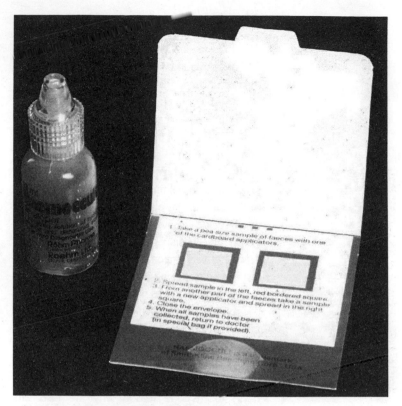

Figure 4.1 A Faecal Occult Blood test (FOBt) kit. The person to be screened receives three folding cards. Two small faecal samples are retrieved and placed on each of the square windows on the card, which is then closed and posted to the screening centre, together with two other identical cards, used on consecutive days. At the centre, hydrogen peroxide (from the small bottle) is dripped onto the windows: if a blue colour appears around the specimen the test is positive.

with a chemical called **guaiac**; when hydrogen peroxide is dripped onto a stool sample, a blue halo may appear around it on the card. If one of the six samples from a screenee develops the halo, the test is deemed positive, leading to a call for a colonoscopy.

guaiac
Chemical impregnated into FOBt card that causes the blue coloration which indicates a positive test when hydrogen peroxide is dripped onto the stool specimen.

What happens after the FOBt?

For all the reasons stated above, a firm diagnosis cannot be made on the basis of the FOBt alone, so a colonoscopy is necessary to discover who, among the ten per cent of screen-positive people, has a cancer. At this examination a cancer may be found, and the patient may be referred to a surgeon. Some cancers will still be at the **malignant polyp** stage, and are treatable simply by removal through the colonoscope. The **endoscopist** may also find (benign) adenomas, which will be removed to prevent them from ever becoming cancers.

Another very important point; while a negative test can be reassuring for the 98 per cent who get such a result, this does not rule out completely the possibility that the person has a cancer; one person in 2,000 who has a negative test has a bowel cancer despite this. The test may have been negative because cancers bleed only intermittently, so the test(s) may have been performed on 'dry days'; this is one reason why the tests are performed on three days rather than just one. So no one whose test is negative should ignore any subsequent symptoms, and should get them checked out by a doctor, in addition for adhering to recommendations for periodic repeat screens.

malignant polyp
An early cancer that has arisen in an adenomatous polyp, and retains the polypoid shape.

endoscopist
The doctor undertaking the colonoscopy. They would also be expert in the use of the gastroscope, which is passed through the mouth to examine the oesophagus, stomach and duodenum.

The outcome of treatment for FOBt-detected cancer

Around 50 per cent of cancers found this way will be at Dukes' stage A (the earliest stage, see Chapter 8), which carries a 95 per cent chance of cure with appropriate treatment. This compares with just ten per cent at Dukes' stage A amongst those who get to a doctor only after symptoms have developed. Furthermore, around 25 per cent of the FOBt screen-detected cancers will be so early in their growth that they are treatable simply by removing them via the colonoscope, compared to just one to two per cent of those presenting with symptoms.

Other methods of mass screening

So far, we have concentrated on the use of the guaiac FOBt and have discussed all the big issues relating to bowel cancer screening as if this were the only method available. In fact, although they haven't been investigated nearly as thoroughly, there are other tests and methods that deserve mention.

Other types of FOBt

Other faecal occult blood tests use different chemical means for detecting blood. One such test can quantify the amount of blood present; as the amount could give a clue to the cause of bleeding and this may have a technical advantage. The test is more complicated to perform and rather more expensive, so it is not seen as a potential mass screening test. Another sort of occult blood test exploits the new technology of **monoclonal antibodies**. These tests, known as **immunoassays**, have the theoretical advantage of testing positive only to human blood, thereby decreasing the false positive rate, and with it the anxiety and cost associated with false positive results. So far, however, these tests have not proven themselves to be more discriminating than the guaiac-based FOBt.

> **myth**
> Colonoscopy sounds horrible and it's bound to hurt.

> **fact**
> It may not sound very inviting, but everything is done to prevent it from being 'horrible'. For a start, if you want it or need it, you will get some very effective – and even pleasant – sedation to make you comfortable; and if you want to, you can usually watch the test in glorious Technicolor on your own small CCTV monitor!

> **monoclonal antibodies (Mab)**
> Proteins made very specifically to find and to fuse with particular target proteins (antigens).

> **immunoassay**
> A test that determines the presence or absence of certain compounds (such as one occurring only in human blood cells) using specific antibodies.

Faecal tumour product tests

It ought to be possible to detect substances other than blood shed into the bowel motions. Theoretically cancer cells shed into the stool should contain proteins which only occur in cancer cells, or at least in larger amounts than in normal cells. **Carcinoembryonic antigen (CEA)** is one such substance, but attempts to use this as a 'stool marker' have failed on technical grounds so far. Some cancer-causing genes (oncogenes), shed into the stool in cancer cells, can be detectable in the faeces. Developing this approach into a practical method would certainly be a major leap forward in screening technology.

carcinoembryonic antigen (CEA)

A protein present in cells, including the bowel epithelium, that is produced in excess in various conditions, including bowel cancer. It escapes into the bloodstream and the faeces, and in excessive amounts may indicate the presence of cancer.

Tumour markers in the blood

A completely different approach is to look for substances released from tumours into the blood (**tumour markers**). Again, CEA has been investigated. When this substance was first discovered in the 1960s it was seen first and foremost as the great hope for screening. However, CEA testing misses a large proportion of early cancers and may be present in increased amounts in the blood of people with other conditions or with no condition at all. The prospect of mass screening using a blood test is seen by many researchers as a more complicated and costly approach than testing the stool.

tumour markers

Substances in bodily fluids, particularly blood, the presence of which suggests the presence of cancer. CEA being one of these.

Endoscopic screening

Endoscopic screening, using the colonoscope or flexible sigmoidoscope, is the other major approach to screening being looked at very actively, particularly in the UK. Colonoscopy, though widely used as a screening tool in the US, applied not as a national public health programme but on an individual *ad hoc* basis, is not seen to be a viable approach in the UK and the rest of Europe or Canada, and will not be discussed further here.

Flexible sigmoidoscopy (Flexiscope) which uses a 60 cm flexible 'telescope' to enable examination of the large bowel from the anus to the splenic flexure, is quite a different matter as it is simpler, cheaper and safer. This test is the subject of a major trial in the UK, involving initially 400,000 people.

my experience I was approached by the research team to take part in their trial to test the Flexiscope. I wasn't sure, but if it was going to help other people I was prepared to go along. In fact it was dead easy: the staff were so nice and did all they could to help me avoid embarrassment. I was really pleased the test was normal, and will tell my friends to have it if the research shows it's a good thing.

The principle here is not just early detection of cancer, but the identification and removal of adenomas before they can develop into cancer. The test is performed by inserting a 60 cm scope, with a camera at the tip, into the rectum, and passing it up through the sigmoid colon to the splenic flexure (see Figure 4.2). This whole segment of the bowel has the highest incidence of adenomas and cancer. Adenomas develop mostly between the ages of 55 and 65, so performing the test in this period ought to give the best chance of cancer prevention. It is performed as an outpatient, and the only **bowel preparation** required is a simple enema after arrival at the hospital. The test is very safe, and there has been only a small proportion of screenees in the trial who have found the experience unpleasant. Most adenomas

bowel preparation
Cleaning of the inside of the large bowel to allow the best view during endoscopy. Methods include a strong laxative drink (Citramag or Picolax) and cleaning 'from below' using an enema (the norm for flexible sigmoidoscopy).

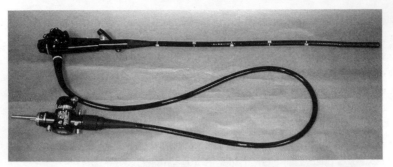

Figure 4.2 A flexible sigmoidoscope ('Flexiscope'). This is a 60 cm long scope; the 'business end' is the straight part at the top, with the white, 10 cm markers on it. This is passed through the anus to allow detailed inspection of the rectum and left side of the colon.

identified are removed at the same time, though larger or multiple adenomas are seen as making a full colonoscopy necessary as they predict that there may be disease beyond the reach of the Flexiscope that would require attention; this is the case for five per cent of those screened.

One very important attribute of this test is that it is likely to be needed just once, at around the age of 60, to have a major effect in cancer prevention, compared to the two-yearly re-testing needed for FOBt. The national trial of this approach should report its results in 2007, making available the evidence necessary to allow decisions about its use in national screening. It might well be that this test would be added into the programme, being performed once on men and women in their late fifties before FOBt is offered at age 60 onwards to give extra assurance.

Selective screening of high risk groups

The FOBt aims to select a smaller group from the wider population for more detailed scrutiny, based on their higher risk of cancer as suggested by the screening test. Another way to define a smaller group is to look at aspects of people that might place them into a **higher risk group** without the need to subject them to any further test. Let's look at these high risk groups.

Family history and cancer risk

Most people are aware that cancer seems to 'run' in some families; certainly there are such families, as we discussed in Chapter 3. Doctors caring for bowel cancer patients are becoming more aware of these family-related risks, and clinics have been set up around the country to look specifically at the care of such families, and to counsel those who are anxious that their family may be carrying some increased risk. Regular colonoscopies and removal of adenomas considerably decreases the cancer risk in people with an inherited increased risk.

Inflammatory bowel disease

Ulcerative colitis and, to a lesser extent, Crohn's disease can increase an individual's bowel cancer risk. This was discussed in Chapter 3. People who have had ulcerative colitis for ten years or more, especially those with extensive involvement of

higher risk group
A subgroup of a population who have in common a raised risk for a particular condition.

myth
If cancer is in the family, that's it: there's nothing that's going to stop me getting cancer, so I'm not having them poke me around for nothing. I'll just take my chances, thank you very much.

fact
If you are having regular colonoscopies, you actually have less risk of getting bowel cancer than the rest of the population. That's because removing benign adenomas reduces the risk – no adenomas, no progression to cancer.

my experience
When I was diagnosed with mild ulcerative colitis, my best friend told me that his cousin had died of cancer because he had UC. That really put the wind up me, so I asked my specialist. He said that there can be a risk in UC but that it's really only in people with more severe and widespread colitis than I've got, and even then it's only after having it for about ten years. Boy, was I relieved. Just shows you shouldn't always believe your friends!

the colon and rectum, are at particular risk, and should be offered special surveillance.

Most doctors would agree that patients with longstanding, extensive ulcerative colitis should be seen every two years and questioned carefully about any symptoms. They should undergo a colonoscopy and biopsies should be taken from the bowel lining, looking for the tell-tale microscopic signs of 'dysplasia', a change in the appearance of the bowel lining cells which may suggest that cancer could develop in the near future, or may already have occurred elsewhere in the bowel. A finding of dysplasia should lead to cancer-preventive surgery. Complete colonoscopic examination of this patient group, at regular intervals, is practised by many centres looking after colitis patients. This process is often called clinical surveillance.

Summary

Bowel cancer prevention, whether primary or secondary, to prevent premature death, is a laudable aim and one into which much research effort has been, and continues to be, directed. True prevention may require a more complete understanding of the causative factors for the disease, while success in screening and secondary prevention demands better tests, uptake by those at most risk, and sufficient application of human and financial resources. These approaches certainly offer a very good opportunity to make major inroads into the death rate from bowel cancer.

CHAPTER

5

The symptoms of bowel cancer and when to go to the doctor

We tend to think of normal health and disease as being quite clearly separable, but often this is not the case. The onset of the symptoms of bowel cancer is a very good example of how ill health can creep up without being very obvious at first. Little wonder that on average there are about six months between the onset of the symptoms of bowel cancer and going to the doctor. Perhaps the main reason is that the symptoms of bowel cancer overlap with those of more common, less serious problems such as piles.

Before we can say what symptoms should take us along to the doctor, we need to understand a little of how these symptoms might develop, and the grouping together of symptoms that should trigger attention. The first thing to say may come as a surprise to those blessed with 'clockwork' bowel function – there is a great variety and range of normal function between different people. Furthermore, we all get aches, pains and other symptoms that we blame on our stomach or bowel; for some of us these are regular and sometimes very disabling though usually not due to any identifiable or serious underlying cause. Bleeding is common, with 20 per cent of people asked in a Portsmouth survey admitting to noticing blood in their stool in the previous year.

One of the aims of this chapter is to provide sensible guidelines on when to consult a doctor about symptoms that could be due to bowel cancer. First, we should try to define 'normal bowel function' so that we can see how bowel cancer symptoms might develop and differ from our normal pattern.

What is 'normal' bowel function?

myth

If you don't do a number two every day there's something wrong with you.

fact

That's an old wives' tale and the reason so many people now in their seventies and eighties were given castor oil or other laxatives every day throughout childhood. There is simply no such thing as a single 'normal' bowel habit – people vary enormously in their frequency and timing of visits to the toilet.

A survey of a random sample of south Londoners aged 55 years and older revealed a remarkable variation in beliefs and attitudes about the bowels. Like all surveys, its results cannot be taken as certain truth, but it does illustrate the range of function that different people accept as normal, and therefore may help us to know what to think about our own bowel habit. Men reported moving their bowels more often than women; two-thirds of the men and just over half of the women moved their bowels once daily. About one-fifth of men and one-tenth of women had regular motions, but only every few days, sometimes separated by a week or more. A large majority of both sexes reported that their bowel patterns were regular. Most respondents were satisfied by their bowel frequency; only 11 per cent felt that their bowels did not open often enough and just three per cent thought that their bowels opened too frequently. For about one in seven respondents, satisfactory results were achieved after some effort, habitually using something to keep their bowels regular. Two-thirds of the whole group had used 'over the counter' laxatives at some time, and over half paid regular attention to their diet to improve their bowel function.

This all goes to show that bowel habits can vary widely and why it is not possible or useful to try to define too narrowly what is 'normal'.

The important symptoms of bowel cancer

The following list highlights persistent or recurrent symptoms to look out for. These include:

✧ a change in bowel habit (change in frequency, or a tendency towards **looser motions**)

✧ **blood** and/or mucus with the motions

✧ abdominal pain

✧ **tenesmus**, a constant feeling of incomplete emptying of the bowel

✧ general symptoms – weight loss, **tiredness**, loss of appetite, etc.

The differences between 'normal' bowel function and the symptoms of bowel cancer

The presence of bowel cancer may make itself known in several ways, depending on its location in the bowel and its state of advance. Perhaps the best way to understand the symptoms that may

myth
Everybody gets tummy upsets, and bleeding is very common. So there's no need to bother the doctor, and anyway, it's so embarrassing to talk to a near stranger about your bowels.

fact
First sentence – true. However, don't take your health for granted. If you get these symptoms for more than a few weeks, let your doctor decide whether they matter or not.

loose motions
Funny word, 'loose'. This just means anything other than 'formed' – which means the stool is firm enough to maintain its shape.

tenesmus
An important symptom – even with regular 'good' bowel movements a person is left with the feeling of a full rectum.

tiredness
We all think we feel tired a lot! Here it might be a feature of anaemia, which makes getting enough oxygen around the body less efficient.

myth
If you haven't got any symptoms you can't have bowel cancer.

fact
You certainly can. Most cancers have usually been there for months or years before they produce symptoms, so it is no surprise that many patients are beyond cure by the time they get to the doctor. The simple message is that you should not delay further once you recognize the possible warning symptoms.

anaemia
'Thinning' of the blood – a shortage of red blood cells – that can be due to various causes, but here is due to blood loss from the bowel sufficient that the body cannot replace it fast enough to prevent anaemia.

develop is to apply what we have already discussed about the anatomy and function of the bowel. The bowel is a hollow tube containing faeces that is liquid as it enters the caecum (first part of the colon) and gradually thickens as water is absorbed while it makes its way to the rectum. If a growth from the inner lining of that tube gradually enlarges, what trouble can it cause to warn us of its presence? There are two main local effects of the tumour that may cause symptoms which should engage our attention:

✧ it can shed blood or mucus into the faeces, resulting in an altered appearance and consistency of the stool
✧ it can narrow the bowel, causing a change in stool character, and perhaps cramping pain due to stronger bowel contractions to push faeces through the narrower channel.

A bowel tumour may also have general effects, such as:

✧ symptoms due to **anaemia** (as a result of blood loss), such as tiredness and lethargy
✧ weight loss, decreased appetite.

Although there are no set patterns, symptoms also vary depending on the segment of bowel affected.

Cancer of the right colon (caecum and ascending colon)

This often produces symptoms later than tumours further downstream. Blood or mucus shed into the right colon usually becomes mixed in with the stool and altered by bacterial action before getting to the rectum, so obvious blood may not be seen in the motion. If there is a significant loss, blood partially degraded by bacteria may darken the stool, perhaps making it maroon-coloured or even darker. Most commonly, there is no obvious change in the appearance of the motions and the only way to tell whether blood is being lost in the stools is to check for anaemia with a simple blood examination, or to check the stool with a chemical test for occult (hidden) blood (faecal occult blood testing). Tiredness due to chronic blood loss may be the first symptom of right-sided colon cancer; it can even induce angina (heart pain) if the anaemia results in decreased oxygen delivery to the heart muscle. If unexplained anaemia is found particularly in a person over the age of 40, the possibility of colon cancer should be considered.

my experience

I enjoy my golf – always have – so I was very disappointed when I started to get puffed pulling my cart down the back nine: I thought I was getting past it, and would have to pack It in. Then I saw some blood in the toilet, so I went to the doctor. To cut a long story short, I was anaemic due to a bowel cancer. Since I've had it cut out, I'm back on the course with my pals, and taking their money off them as regular as ever!

Change in bowel habit may be minimal or absent in right-sided colon cancer. This is most likely due to the liquid nature of the faeces in this part of the colon, which allows it to find its way through a narrowed channel. It usually takes a large mass in the caecum or right colon to cause any obstacle to the flow of faeces. Thus, the tumour's presence may go unnoticed for some time. Sometimes, and in the absence of any other symptoms, a right-sided cancer can be felt by the patient as a lump through the front of the abdomen.

Cancer of the sigmoid colon and rectum

Bleeding is the most common symptom of cancer of the sigmoid colon and rectum. The blood may be well mixed into the stool or, especially in low-lying tumours, may appear as streaks on the surface of the stool, identical to the pattern seen with piles.

Change of bowel habit is a prominent symptom. The bowel loses its normal timetable, with periods of constipation alternating with diarrhoea. Diarrhoea may occur because solid stool may not easily get past the tumour. Narrowing of the sigmoid colon may cause abdominal cramping pain. Later the bowel may become completely blocked, causing severe pains, reminiscent of childbirth to female patients, distension of the abdomen and, eventually, vomiting.

An important symptom of rectal cancer is tenesmus, the constant feeling of a full rectum. The brain interprets the presence of a tumour mass as stool but it cannot be passed. This feeling causes frequent visits to the toilet, the sensation of incomplete emptying and straining may only produce some bloody mucus.

A more constant pain in the back or sacral area, not related to bowel motions, can result from the invasion of other structures outside the rectum. This is a later symptom and usually signifies more advanced disease.

Cancer of the transverse and left colon

Tumours in this part of the bowel, lying between the two areas described above, may cause symptoms from both the above-mentioned symptom patterns.

Rarer symptoms of bowel cancer, due to advanced tumours spreading outside the bowel, include:

✧ pain on passing urine, perhaps with air (**pneumaturia**) or small particles of stool (looking like tea leaves) noticed in the urine. This is due to the tumour invading the bladder, followed by leakage of stool and flatus

✧ passage of stool through the vagina due to a tumour penetrating the back of the vagina.

Both symptoms are very distressing, and although it might be thought that such problems could only be due to cancer, they can also be due to other, non-malignant bowel conditions, especially **diverticular disease**.

When should you go to the doctor?

The south London survey mentioned earlier showed that one-third of the respondents had consulted a doctor about their bowels at least once at some time prior to receiving the questionnaire, and nearly half of those aged 65–74 had done so. The most common reasons for consulting a doctor were, in descending order, constipation, pain, bleeding or diarrhoea. These

pneumaturia
You may hear the doctor use this word, literally describing air in the urine.

diverticular disease
A very common disorder of the colon, usually the sigmoid, in which small 'bubbles' form on its outer surface, sometimes leading to complications, including leakage of faeces into the bladder or vagina.

were, by design of the survey, people without cancer, so the investigation of their symptoms did not lead to a diagnosis of bowel cancer.

As any of these symptoms can be due to less sinister conditions, there is a tendency for many of us to put off 'bothering the doctor'. It is little wonder that, on average, it takes six months for people to become sufficiently concerned by their symptoms to get round to seeking advice.

What, then, are the symptoms that justify a visit to the doctor and how long should they be present before the time comes to ring up the surgery and make the appointment?

◈ *Bleeding* – Blood, especially if mixed with the stool or if dark in colour, should be a signal to see the doctor. Although bright blood only on the toilet paper is less worrying, it is nevertheless best checked out, especially amongst those beyond 50 years of age.

◈ *Change in bowel habit* – This important symptom may be minimal: someone with a long-standing habit of passing one bowel action each morning may find that they have to make a second visit before leaving for work. For others the change may be more obvious. In any case, an unexplained change going on for more than a few weeks needs attention.

◈ *Pain* – Lots of us get abdominal pains and in most cases it is not an indication of cancer. However, cramping pain, especially if it is persistent or recurrent, perhaps associated with other symptoms, may be due to a constricting growth in the bowel. When in doubt, check it out.

Q I had a gippy tummy for six months before I got the courage to go to the doctor, and sure enough it turned out I had bowel cancer. Does it matter that I left it so long?

A Believe it or not, you left it no longer than the average. As far as we can tell, it doesn't make any great difference, though that should certainly not discourage people from seeking medical advice early if they are concerned about themselves. The big difference comes when we make the diagnosis before symptoms start, by carrying out a screening test. But that's another story, as you will remember from Chapter 4.

✧ *Tenesmus* – As explained above, a constant feeling of incomplete emptying of the rectum is an important symptom of rectal cancer. If this symptom is present, it needs to be looked into.

What should the doctor do?

Since the year 2000, general practitioners have been using very specific recommendations from the National Health Service about which symptoms should trigger referral to hospital for a specialist opinion. And not only that – there are arrangements that ensure that any patient referred using these guidelines is seen by a specialist within **two weeks**. The doctor simply fills in a form and faxes it to the hospital and the process swings into action. One of the following referral criteria for any adult patient, whatever their age, must be met for the doctor to use this mechanism:

> **the 'two week rule'**
> This has led successfully to much quicker hospital referral. It applies to all sorts of cancer, not just bowel cancer. There are rules now regulating the speed with which patients are investigated and treated. This will be described later.

✧ definitely palpable lump in right side of the abdomen
✧ definitely palpable lump inside the rectum
✧ rectal bleeding with change in bowel habit to more frequent defaecation or looser stools (or both) persistent over six weeks
✧ iron deficiency anaemia (blood count less than ten in men, or less than 11 in women after the menopause) without obvious cause
✧ rectal bleeding persistently without anal symptoms (soreness, discomfort, itching, lumps, prolapse, pain).

my experience

I started bleeding, so I went straight to the doctor, like you're supposed to. The doctor gave me the fright of my life when she stuck her finger up my behind and told me she thought I had cancer. I knew it took forever to get to see someone down the hospital, and what does the government do about it? But Dr Webster said there was a new rule, and that the hospital had to see me within two weeks. And they did. I was frightened when they told me that my doctor had got it right, and that I'd need an operation. But at least I was spared the dreadful anxiety I would have had if I'd had to hang around for weeks before even getting to the outpatients. So now, thank goodness, we can just get on with it.

Summary

The symptoms of bowel cancer may creep up gradually, and may seem to be of little consequence at first. The main message is: unexplained bowel symptoms that persist for six weeks, especially in the middle-aged and elderly, need to be reported to the doctor. Let the doctor decide whether the symptoms warrant specialist assessment. If they do, the NHS ensures you are seen at the hospital quickly, cutting down as much as possible the anxiety that goes with not knowing whether you might have bowel cancer.

CHAPTER

6

Seeking medical help

The previous chapter dealt with the symptoms as they make themselves apparent to the patient before going to the doctor and suggested how the doctor might begin to weigh them up. This chapter deals with the consequences of deciding to make that visit – the road from the GP's surgery to the hospital outpatient department, the investigations that might follow, leading up to a diagnosis. We will consider treatment in later chapters.

Visiting the family doctor

The family doctor has several tasks including:

✧ obtaining an accurate picture of the problem from the patient
✧ deciding on a group of possible diagnoses, hopefully including the correct one

✧ deciding whether they can manage the problem, or whether the patient should be referred to a specialist

✧ deciding which specialist is most appropriate, if referral seems necessary

✧ taking any immediate steps needed for the comfort and safety of the patient.

The family doctor, unlike the hospital doctor, is likely to have met the patient before and will know them to some extent. This is very important when it comes to assessing the significance of the symptoms. Hearing about the bleeding or about the change of bowel habit, alarm bells might start ringing, and on the story alone the doctor should be coming up with a list of diagnostic possibilities that might include bowel cancer. Next the doctor should examine the patient, including feeling inside the rectum with a rubber glove. The problem arises, however, of whether all patients with these symptoms should be referred to the hospital. Family doctors see lots of patients with minor 'tummy upsets' and small amounts of bleeding, and referral of every one is unnecessary and would certainly overwhelm the hospital. Bright red bleeding only noticed on the toilet paper (likely to be due to piles), or diarrhoea in more than one household member at the same time (likely to be due to a stomach bug) can be dealt with, at least initially, by the family doctor. However, unless there is some easy and confident explanation, especially in the over-fifties, referral for consultant examination and investigation is appropriate. On average, however, there is a six month delay between onset of symptoms and going to the doctor in patients with bowel cancer. This delay, generated by the patient and the family doctor, is partly due to the considerable overlap between the symptoms of bowel cancer and those of harmless conditions such as piles.

Hospital referral is usually to a surgeon. However, sometimes the diagnosis will be far from obvious, the family doctor simply feeling that there may be something seriously wrong but not knowing what or where. The patient may be vaguely unwell, for example with weight loss and anaemia, in which case the referral might be to a general physician or a specialist in the care of the elderly. If the patient is anaemic they might be sent first to a blood specialist to check out why. If the family doctor feels that a surgical referral is appropriate, ideally this should be to a surgeon with a special interest in bowel disorders, as they are most likely to be able to offer the widest range of specialist procedures needed to treat the various types and stages of bowel cancer.

Referral to the hospital

Patients with symptoms that are strongly linked with bowel cancer should have been referred under the NHS 'two week rule' (see previous chapter), but in others there may not have been sufficient suspicion of the possible diagnosis, so that routine referral may have occurred.

Diagnosis using appropriate investigations, discussion of the diagnosis with the patient and the family doctor, and deciding on appropriate treatment are the main tasks of the hospital specialist. As has been the case since the dawn of medicine, the process still begins with careful history taking.

Taking the medical history

history taking
Used medically this refers to the careful process of collecting a full picture of the development and present character of any symptoms, and getting details of the patient's general health, social habits, medical past, and any family medical history that might be relevant.

The word **history** in this context relates to the careful recording by the doctor of the presenting symptoms and other relevant past or current medical problems. Although the referral letter from the family doctor will have briefly outlined the symptoms, the specialist will ask the patient to tell the story again. This will not only allow the surgeon's diagnostic thoughts to begin to tick over, it will also allow them to begin to get to know the patient and their insight into the problem. This will be very important when it comes to discussing the diagnosis and treatment later. When the patient has told their story, the surgeon will ask some questions, aimed at making the story clearer, focusing on any areas where more information is needed. They will want to know about other health problems, past medical history, about the patient's family and job, and so on. By the time the history has been taken, the surgeon should have gained as clear a picture as possible of the patient and their symptoms; only then will they begin to come to what is known as a **differential diagnosis**, a short list of several possible causes of the symptoms. The next step is to examine the patient.

differential diagnosis
A series of two, three, four main diagnostic possibilities – the short list from which the actual illness will most likely emerge after further examination and investigation.

Physical examination

Although the surgeon may perform a wide-ranging general examination, they will be looking in much more detail at those areas highlighted by the patient's story. Having checked for general signs of anaemia and weight loss, they will examine the abdomen very carefully while the patient lies on their back. The first stage, **inspection**, involves the surgeon looking carefully at the surface of the abdomen to see if there are any obvious swellings. There follows a gentle examination of the abdomen with the palm of the hand (**palpation**). This may reveal a lump in the line of the bowel, or the liver may be enlarged. Next comes **percussion**, in which one hand is placed on the abdomen and the middle finger struck sharply with the tip of the other middle finger. This strange performance is used to gauge the degree of solidity of the structures immediately within the abdomen, below the right hand. If the bowel is full of gas a sound like a drum is heard, while if a solid organ, such as an enlarged liver, or an abnormal amount of fluid is present a dull thud will be heard. (This technique started with the medical student son of a German wine grower who saw his father tapping on his barrels to check the amount of wine inside.) Finally the surgeon may feel it necessary to listen to the activity of the bowel with a stethoscope (**auscultation**), particularly if the story suggests that there might be a partial obstruction of the bowel.

inspection
The first of the classical four stages of abdominal examination. It means – looking! There's lots to see potentially for the well-trained observer.

palpation
Careful feeling, first with the palm of the hand and then with gently probing fingertips.

percussion
Tapping of the abdomen to distinguish gas from liquid from solid tissue inside – easy when you know how ...

auscultation
The process of listening to the abdomen using a stethoscope. If there is bowel obstruction the usual rather dull and infrequent sounds of the fluid and gas moving along the bowel during its muscular contractions are replaced by louder, more frequent, tinkling notes as the sound bounces around – almost echoes – in the gas within a distended bowel.

my experience

I was dreading the examination. I couldn't see what the surgeon was about to do because I was lying on my side facing away from her. Thank goodness she didn't do anything without telling me first. It was difficult to relax when the finger went in, but she told me it was only like 'passing a stool backwards'! I suppose that's right, but it still felt weird. She warned me that I would feel like going to the loo when she pumped air in through the telescope to help her see, but she was able to reassure me that I was not about to shower her because she could see at first hand that my rectum was empty!

digital rectal examination (DRE)
Again, much to be learned from this. The doctor who omits the DRE in a case that later turns out to be a low rectal cancer may miss the diagnosis.

mobility
A very important item to check. If a tumour moves easily over the underlying tissues in the pelvis, it is said to be 'freely mobile'; if it moves a bit, but does not feel so free, it is 'tethered'; and if the *patient* moves when you push just the tumour, it is 'fixed'. These are the ways that surgeons had to check for spread of the tumour beyond the bowel wall and into surrounding tissues and organs until just 25 years ago, when scanners were invented, and revolutionized this aspect of rectal cancer assessment.

rigid sigmoidoscope
Invented in the late nineteenth century, and still going. A simple metal tube with a light at the business end and a lens at the surgeon's end, it gives a fair view of the bowel lining up to 25 cm from the anus, well beyond the top of the rectum – a technological miracle in 1890!

The next part of the examination is done with the patient lying on their left side with the knees bent up towards the chest. There are two main parts to this examination:

1 Digital examination

This involves the doctor inserting their gloved index finger into the rectum **(digital rectal examination (DRE))**. This may be an embarrassing experience for the patient, who may also expect it to be painful. If he or she can relax (easily said!) the muscles of the anal canal are less likely to resist the doctor's finger, making the examination less uncomfortable. Having applied a little lubricant jelly to the glove, the doctor will insert it gently into the lower rectum via the anus. The lining of the bowel can be felt quite easily: if there is a tumour within reach of the finger this will be felt as a firm lump, perhaps with a hollowed-out, ulcerated centre. The rectal wall is normally quite mobile on the underlying tissues, but an advanced cancer that has invaded through the bowel wall to involve tissues outside will feel much less **mobile** than the surrounding normal bowel. Around 75 per cent of rectal cancers are within reach of the examining finger. On extraction, the surgeon will examine the glove for tell-tale signs of blood or mucus suggestive of a tumour or other abnormality.

2 Sigmoidoscopy

This is direct visual examination of the lining of the bowel using a **rigid sigmoidoscope**. This is a rigid metal or plastic tube, 1.5 cm in diameter and 25 cm long that can reach to the top of the rectum and beyond. The tube is hollow and has a glass lens attached at the outer end to allow the

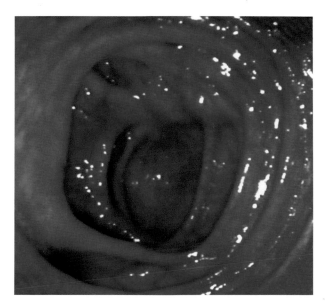

Plate 1 Normal appearance of a colon as seen through a colonoscope. Looking directly along the colon, the concentric rings are folds in the mucosa.

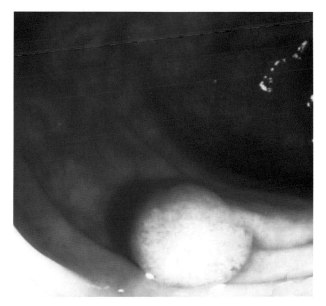

Plate 2 An adenoma in the colon as seen through a colonoscope. The smooth sphere below has the typical benign appearance.

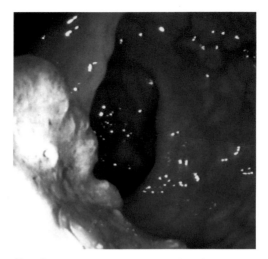

Plate 3 A cancer in the colon as seen through a colonoscope. The tumour, on the left, is irregular and ulcerated. The appearance could be due to nothing else.

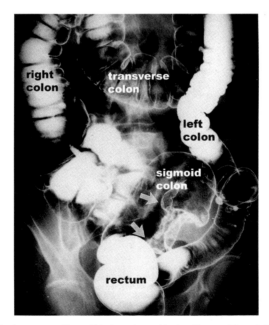

Plate 4 A barium enema X-ray. This is performed by instilling a white solution of barium sulphate via the anus, followed by air to facilitate coating of the bowel wall with barium. This allows the otherwise invisible bowel to be seen on an X-ray. The anatomy is clearly seen here; in the sigmoid colon, between the two arrows, an irregular narrow segment can be seen. Known to doctors as an 'apple core lesion', this has the typical appearance of a cancer.

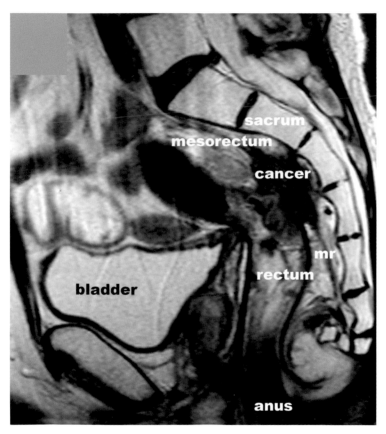

Plate 5 Magnetic resonance (MR) scan. MR allows doctors to examine in great detail the anatomy and pathology in the patient. Here you can see a front-to-back cross section of the pelvis in a man with rectal cancer. The tumour can be seen growing backwards into the mesorectum and threatening to involve the bone at the back of the pelvis (sacrum). The scan has therefore highlighted the need for pre-operative chemoradiotherapy to try to shrink the tumour away from the sacrum before surgery.

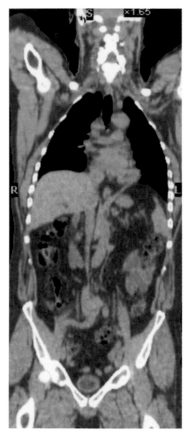

Plate 6 Computerized tomography (CT) scan. The scanner revolves around the patient – like a satellite circling the globe – collecting X-ray information that is used by a computer to display as cross sections of the body. Most pictures are horizontal sections, but here you see a vertical section that shows everything from the neck to the upper thighs. When the hundreds of sections are viewed sequentially an enormous amount of information is available for diagnosis and treatment planning.

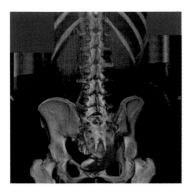 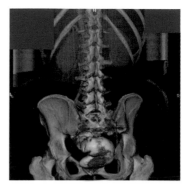

Plate 7 The frontiers of CT examination. These two extraordinary pictures show what is becoming possible with CT imaging. In **(a)** a back view of the chest, abdomen and pelvis are seen, looking extremely like a real skeleton. By 'subtracting' the back of the pelvis **(b)**, the anatomy of the rectum can be revealed. In time this technology will allow 'virtual surgery' – surgeons will be able to work through a difficult operation beforehand using computer simulation.

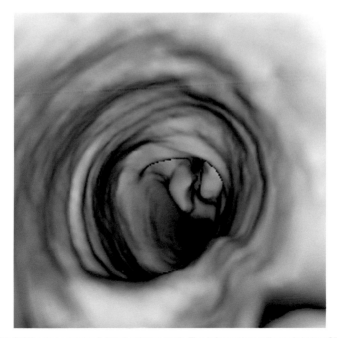

Plate 8 CT colonography ('virtual colonscopy'). The information collected during CT examination can be used by the computer to produce an appearance very much like that seen through a colonoscope (see Plate 2). This is a single frame picture, but by running all the data, the computer permits a 'fly through' view of the entire rectum and colon, seeing any pathology on the way. In this picture the irregular outline of a cancer is seen in the distance.

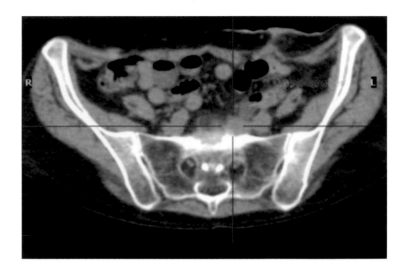

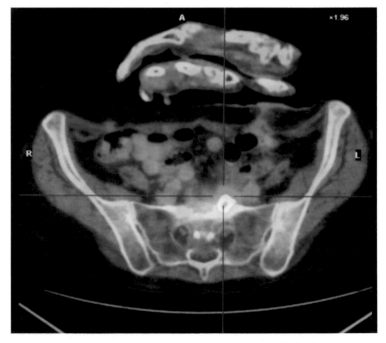

Plate 9 Positron emission tomography, used with simultaneous CT. **(a)** shows a horizontal cross section of the pelvis in a CT scan. The 'cross wires' indicate an abnormal shadow, but is it a recurrent cancer? **(b)** shows the combined CT and PET scans strongly indicate that it is a recurrent cancer, as the PET shows up the otherwise anonymous grey CT abnormality as a bright yellow 'hot spot'.

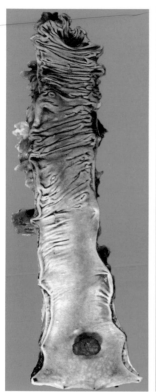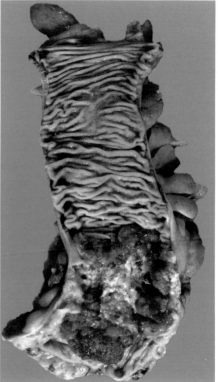

Plate 10 Naked eye appearance of rectal cancer. These two specimens have been taken from rectal resections where the removed bowel has been opened vertically to reveal mucosal lining and cancer. **(a)** shows a small, early stage polypoid cancer and **(b)** shows a larger, fungating advanced cancer.

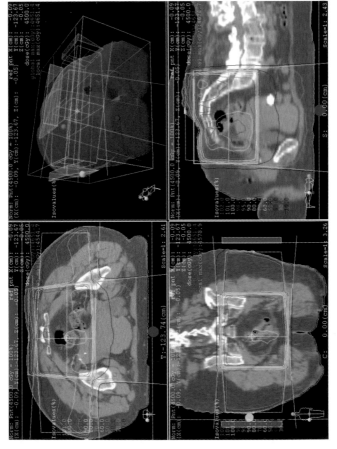

Plate 11 CT scans for planning radiotherapy dose and volume. Every pelvis is a different shape; these scans aid calculation of the most effective dose to the tumour while minimizing damaging irradiation of surrounding normal structures.

surgeon to view through it. Built into the lens attachment is a side tube and small rubber bulb to allow air to be introduced to inflate the rectum gently, making it easier to examine. A light source is also attached to illuminate the inside of the bowel.

Just as with the digital examination, the patient may be anxious at the thought of this procedure. Insertion of the instrument through the anus is not painful. As it is advanced along the rectum and air is introduced into the bowel, the patient may have a sudden feeling of needing to empty the bowel. Sometimes the air escapes from the rectum around the scope, causing further embarrassment to the patient, though the surgeon knows that this is a regular occurrence in this situation and will hopefully try to allay the patient's worries.

The normal lining of the bowel is a yellowish pink colour; the surface is shiny and the minute blood vessels under the mucosa are visible. As the scope is inserted further, the surgeon may see blood or mucus in the bowel, a strongly suspicious sign of a tumour at a higher level. A tumour coming into vision looks very different from the normal mucosa: it may be a discrete lump or a constricting ring. The surface is darker, irregular and may be bleeding. If possible the scope will be pushed gently past the tumour to check its dimensions. The surgeon may pass a special long pair of **forceps** through the sigmoidoscope to snip off a small piece of the lump (a **biopsy**) so that the pathologist can examine it to confirm the diagnosis.

Biopsy is painless: the patient is usually not aware that this is happening. Sometimes, instead of the usual rigid scope, the surgeon will use a

forceps

Instrument that takes a small sample of tissue for examination by the pathologist in order to make a diagnosis.

biopsy

A sample of tissue taken surgically or with a long pair of forceps, which the pathologist can use to make a confident diagnosis.

longer, flexible fibreoptic sigmoidoscope at the routine out-patient visit. This has the advantage of reaching up into the descending colon, thus being able to examine it directly and to biopsy a greater proportion of tumours.

Having completed these examinations the surgeon will often have a clearer idea of the problem. Further investigations will depend on what information is already to hand from the history and examination. There are three main scenarios:

1 **A tumour has been seen through sigmoidoscope**. The surgeon is likely to tell the patient that a growth may be present, pending pathological confirmation, and that an operation is likely to be needed. They will arrange several investigations. First there will be either a colonoscopy or a barium enema X-ray (see page 84) to check the state of the rest of the bowel, as there is a three per cent chance that there is a second cancer elsewhere, known as a **synchronous cancer**. Scans will be arranged to look in more detail at the primary tumour and to check for any distant spread. All these tests will be described in detail later in this chapter.

2 **A tumour has not been seen but suspicions are strong**. Based on the findings so far the surgeon will arrange further investigation, either a colonoscopy or a barium enema, in this case to look for a primary tumour as well as checking the whole of the bowel. Most probably further discussion and any scanning will be reserved until the patient returns for a further outpatient visit after these investigations.

synchronous (Greek 'same time') cancer
The name for that second tumour in the three per cent that have had one cancer identified at initial diagnosis. A second tumour occurring at a later date is **metachronous** (Greek 'after-time').

3 The surgeon concludes that there is not sufficient suspicion to perform any further investigation. There are patients in whom outpatient investigation was needed, but in whom the surgeon is happy not to go further. This might, for instance, be the case in a young patient – in whom cancer would be unlikely anyway – who has complained only of fresh blood on the toilet paper, and who has obvious haemorrhoids on examination.

Special investigations

Colonoscopy

This procedure involves the insertion of a long flexible black tube (colonoscope) to examine the mucosa of the whole colon and rectum (see Plates 1, 2 and 3). It has two advantages over a barium enema X-ray – it is more efficient at finding very small benign adenomas and cancers and it is possible to take biopsies and to remove adenomas at the same time.

Bowel preparation is needed so that the bowel wall can be examined easily and completely. This involves taking a strong laxative at home the day before the examination.

my experience

I was quite concerned about the colonoscopy and hadn't given the 'bowel preparation' a single thought. The idea is to clean the inside of the bowel to give the doctor a perfect view. Sure it was! I took the medicine at home the day before and spent quite a few hours in and out of the toilet. And crumbs, did it make me thirsty. I suppose it was all the water I was losing through my back passage. 'Well done,' said the doctor the next day as he viewed my insides. So I said: 'Sure, I feel well done!'. But all in a good cause: he was able to give me the all clear.

On arrival at the hospital the patient will be laid on their left side and then usually they will be given a sedative injection. The tip of the instrument is inserted through the anus, and the inside of the rectum is immediately visible on the TV monitor. The colonoscopist is able to control the gentle advance of the scope by manipulating two controls. In the average case the scope will reach all the way to the caecum in about 15 to 20 minutes, though if the scope comes up to a very narrowed area it will not be possible to proceed further. The lining of the bowel will be examined particularly carefully as the scope is gently pulled back. If a tumour is seen, a biopsy will be taken to confirm the diagnosis.

The patient rests in the department for a short while after the examination, after which they can go home, accompanied by a relative or friend, a necessary precaution after having been sedated.

Barium enema X-ray

barium enema X-ray
The first examination that allowed anyone to see the inside of the bowel. Still going, but fading fast as colonoscopy takes over.

contrast medium
The name for any fluid or gas injected into the body to help see things in X-rays (by 'contrasting' with tissues around it).

This investigation is used much less these days, and mainly in hospitals where colonoscopy services are less readily available.

Normally the bowel cannot be seen on X-ray pictures as the rays pass straight through it. The principle behind a **barium enema X-ray** is that by introducing a solution of barium sulphate (the **contrast medium**) into the bowel which shows up on the X-ray pictures, the anatomy becomes visible, so any abnormalities can be noted (see Plate 4). Barium sulphate looks rather like, and has the consistency of, single cream. This is run into the rectum through a soft rubber tube and by tipping and turning the patient it is possible to get the barium to pass around the whole rectum and colon. By introducing some air as well (**double contrast barium enema**) the inside surface of the bowel becomes coated with a very thin layer of the barium solution so that surface detail is shown more clearly. The whole examination usually takes around 30 minutes; it may be a little uncomfortable, mainly due to distension of the bowel with air, but it should not be painful.

On X-raying the abdomen the bowel and the fine details of its lining show up very clearly. Any lumps or narrowings can be detected. Lumps as small as a few millimetres in diameter can be seen. After the examination, the patient will pass barium from the bowel for a day or two, making the faeces white. The radiologist will not be able to give an immediate verdict on the examination, preferring to spend some time at the end of the session examining the pictures prior to writing a report for the surgeon.

> **double contrast barium enema**
> Adding air to the barium increases massively the sensitivity of the examination to see small tumours. With 'single contrast' smaller tumours were lost in a sea of whiteness.

Cross sectional imaging

Today we have some very powerful diagnostic tools available to us; amongst them are the various forms of **cross-sectional imaging**. The principle is that a large amount of information is collected using a scanner, after which a computer uses the data to construct hundred of cross-sectional images, effectively slicing the patient very thinly – sometimes every few millimetres, so that the internal organs and any diseases affecting them can be viewed in incredible detail. These technologies began to enter service less than a generation ago and have profoundly altered patient management. The four methods, MRI, CT, USS and PET, are described below.

> **cross-sectional imaging**
> This has swept the field – it is taking over rapidly from most of the older imaging techniques.

Magnetic resonance imaging (MRI, or MR)

magnetic resonance imaging (MRI)
This is the technology of choice for detailed examination of a rectal cancer.

Magnetic resonance imaging (MRI) is transforming the management of rectal cancer. The technology involves placing the patient in a very strong magnetic field rather than using X-rays. With the most modern machines the radiologist is able to produce highly detailed cross-sectional images in three planes – horizontally, vertically, both from side to side (coronal view) and from front to back (sagittal view). The pictures allow the surgeon to visualize very precisely the shape of a rectal tumour, its extent and its anatomical relationship to surrounding tissues and organs (see Plate 5). This allows decisions to be taken on the type of surgery and, importantly, whether the patient should undergo radiotherapy before the operation to 'shrink' the tumour. In the few patients in whom other organs (bladder, prostate, uterus, small bowel or sacrum [the pelvic tail bone]) are seen to be infiltrated, the surgeon can plan appropriately extended surgery. This is a far cry from just a generation ago when all the surgeon had to go on was the information transmitted via the **'educated finger'**.

the 'educated finger'
Surgeons pride themselves on what they can tell with their gloved(!) finger – and it was all they had until well into the late twentieth century. It is still extremely important in helping the surgeon literally to 'get a feel' of the problem. But modern imaging has become the standard.

From the patient's viewpoint the most obvious element of the scanner is a vertical round opening, about three feet across, through which they are delivered on a couch into a tube around which the magnet revolves. They will spend several minutes 'inside', and while the scan is happening there is a lot of noise. A few patients particularly troubled by claustrophobia may not be able to go through with this examination.

The MR scan was quite different from having an ordinary X-ray. As I lay on a rather narrow couch, I was rolled into a tunnel; I had voice contact with the radiographer and a mirror above my head let me see past my feet to the outside. I was warned that it would be noisy when the machine was turned on, and for good reason: it sounded like being in *Dr Who*! Funnily enough I actually dropped off to sleep as the machine made its electronic noises, but I woke up with a jump when it stopped.

Computerized tomography (CT)

Computerized tomography is an older technology than MRI, and uses X-rays to produce cross-sectional images, usually confined to the horizontal ('axial') plane. As in MRI, the patient passes into an opening in the machine, but the experience is less likely to cause a problem for the claustrophobic. This type of scan is employed to examine the chest and abdomen as well as the pelvis (see Plates 6 and 7), although MRI is more useful there. In cases of rectal cancer it is used to look for evidence of distant spread, while in colon cancer cases it provides anatomical detail of the primary tumour as well. A recent development in CT scanning is known as **CT colonography**. This ingenious technique can provide information in patients in whom the colonoscope cannot be taken around the bowel (in frail patients or if the colon is too narrow to allow complete visual colonoscopy). It is even possible to get the computer to deliver the X-ray data in a format that mimics the view through the colonoscope (see Plate 8) – hence its alternative name, virtual colonoscopy.

Ultrasound scan (USS)

The **ultrasound scan** involves delivering a beam of sound beyond the audible frequencies

computerized axial tomography
Originally known as 'the CAT scan', today just simply 'the CT'. Excellent all round scan, which came a decade or two before MRI.

CT colonography (CTC)
Computerized magic! The CT can be used to generate pictures that look just like the 3D view up a colonoscope – without invading the patient!

ultrasound scan (USS)
The earliest, cheapest and most widely available scanning method. Still very good at examining the liver for secondary spread, and the best test for checking the depth of spread of a small cancer into the wall of the rectum.

into the body via a hand held box ('probe');
tissues of different densities reflect the sound
back differently. The returning sound is converted
by a computer into a 'map' on which the internal
organs and abnormalities within them can be
seen. In patients with bowel cancer ultrasound
scans may be used to check that there are no
metastases in the liver. In some instances a
special ultrasound probe inserted into the rectum
can be used to examine tumours low down in the
rectum.

Positron emission tomography (PET)

Positron emission tomography is the latest
and very useful form of examination that
employs a very mildly radioactive substance (an
radionuclide or isotope) to seek out cancer
tissue, which can then be seen using a detector
and displayed pictorially. The isotope is built into
a type of sugar molecule and is therefore taken
into cells as if it were a food energy source;
overactive cells – in areas of inflammation or
malignancy – take up more of this material and
so are 'hotter' on a scan. The PET scan itself is
rather blurry, like trying to see things in a steamy
room. Recently it has become possible to
perform PET and CT scans simultaneously and
superimpose them, so that we get the
anatomical clarity of the CT helping to locate
much more precisely any hot areas on the PET
(see Plates 9a and 9b).

PET alone is very useful as a supportive scan in
hunting for recurrence anywhere in the body
prior, say, to an operation to remove an
apparently single area of recurrence (not much
use removing one area in the hope of cure if

inoperable cancer is left behind elsewhere). PET/CT has its main use in clarifying the nature of an area of abnormality on a conventional CT or MR scan. Is that grey area on the CT or MR a recurrence (and therefore a potential target for surgery), or just a scar from previous surgery?

This is an important addition to the scanning methods available and has yet fully to find its place.

Pulling it all together

By the time all the information from initial examination and the investigations has been produced, the input of several specialists has occurred. These days in the NHS, every case is discussed at a meeting attended by *all* those specialists before any decisions are made about advice to the patient. In addition to the surgeon, pathologist and radiologist, an oncologist and a **clinical nurse specialist (CNS)** are present to make their specialist input. This whole group is known as the **multidisciplinary team (MDT)** and it meets weekly.

> **Q** Does it really make sense to make all the members of an MDT interrupt their busy schedule every week to sit around and discuss management when it should be pretty obvious to everyone what needs to be done?
>
> **A** It certainly does. It ensures that everyone is fully aware of all aspects of every case, and allows discussion between, say, the surgeon and oncologist that might otherwise be restricted to a quick letter either way.

This is a much better process than the surgeon simply receiving written reports on scans and

clinical nurse specialist (CNS)
Until quite recently CNS only meant 'central nervous system'. In its new role this acronym describes a crucial member of the cancer team, the experienced nurse whose main responsibility is to support and inform their cancer patients and to be easily available for guidance and help at all times. Just as with the new technologies, the participation of a clinical nurse specialist has become the standard of care.

multidisciplinary team (MDT)
Another fairly new 'invention', but undoubtedly a very powerful tool in making cancer care as good as we can get it. Every professional involved in the care of any cancer patient has to meet together every week to check progress and discuss options.

other tests, and then having to introduce further delay by sending the patient to the oncologist another day. Together the MDT agrees a plan of action that can be put to the patient at their next outpatient visit.

This outpatient visit to discuss treatment options is obviously very important and we will try to cover its nature and progression carefully here. For a start, it is best if a relative or close friend comes along to provide moral support and to act as a second pair of ears to take in the often complex information to be imparted. The CNS should ideally be present at this meeting to play their key role in offering further clarification and support after the surgeon has left the room and to act as the immediate point of contact (by phone) after the patient has gone home in case they have any further queries or concerns.

> **my experience**
>
> I was so pleased to have a clinical nurse specialist present whenever I was seeing the surgeon or the oncologist. I'm sorry to say that I felt that with the surgeon I couldn't open up on all my fears about my future, and he seemed to be in and out so quickly. My nurse, Tollie, was so kind and reassuring, and she was always there to talk on the phone when I needed her and was so good at explaining everything. 'Half knowing' things just made me more afraid; she filled in the gaps and so made me feel more positive.

The professionals should be doing their best to be clear and to try to ease what the patient may find an overwhelming and intimidating experience: they must also ensure that the patient does not feel pressurized into agreeing to a particular course of action during the consultation. They should be the first to acknowledge the patient's need to go away and think it all through with the help of others before treatment is decided. For some patients it is easy to assimilate the information and to decide on the way forward. If this is the case, the surgeon may be able to offer a date for admission there and then, making the difficult period before treatment easier to cope with as there is at least a timetable agreed.

Emergency hospital admission

Up to 30 per cent of all bowel cancer patients present as emergency cases, having developed one of the major complications (bowel obstruction or perforation). Yet around three-quarters of these will have visited their family doctor at an earlier stage with symptoms that only now can be seen as having been warning signs that were not picked up on. This highlights the difficulty sometimes in recognizing the potentially serious nature of bowel symptoms that overlap with those of less serious but more common conditions.

Obstruction of the bowel causes intermittent severe cramping abdominal pain, cessation of bowel action, abdominal distension and vomiting. Perforation of the bowel causes **peritonitis**, characterized by very severe abdominal pain which is constant and made worse by movement and by breathing. Here again there may be vomiting and distension of the abdomen.

In both situations it is usually apparent to the patient and their relatives that he or she is very ill, leading to call-out of the family doctor or the summoning of an ambulance. When the patient arrives at the hospital they will be seen by an Emergency Department doctor. From a rapid

peritonitis
Inflammation of the inside of the abdomen, usually caused by leakage from the bowel, in this case due to the tumour in its wall.

appraisal of the symptoms and findings on examination, it should be possible to reach a diagnosis of bowel obstruction or perforation, though the precise cause can only be suspected at this stage. The doctor may decide that the patient is sufficiently ill to need an intravenous drip before any investigation. Some blood tests will be ordered and X-rays of the abdomen and chest will be performed, hopefully quickly. The X-ray films may show the tell-tale signs of distension of the bowel suggesting obstruction or peritonitis due to perforation. Gas that may have escaped from the bowel will be seen, clinching a diagnosis of perforation.

Having established that one of these diagnoses is likely, the doctor will call the duty surgeon, whose task it will be to decide on further treatment, almost certainly including an operation. Details of these decisions and of the treatment required in these circumstances will be discussed in Chapters 7 and 9.

> **my experience**
>
> When I was taken in by ambulance with really bad pains in my tummy, I knew that something very serious had happened. I'm home now, but my doctors tell me I nearly didn't make it. They had to operate in the middle of the night because I had peritonitis from a burst cancer. If only I had listened to my wife when she told me I should see the doctor about my diarrhoea and weight loss.

Summary

Now we have looked at the various ways in which a patient suspected of having bowel cancer is likely to be cared for in the process of coming to a firm diagnosis. The time has now come to look at the various ways in which the condition can be dealt with, as explained in the next few chapters.

CHAPTER

7

Surgery for bowel cancer

This is the longest chapter in the book. Some might say that this is because two of the authors are surgeons! Perhaps – but it is mainly that surgery is the central element in the management of bowel cancer and will be an abiding experience for the patient and their loved ones. We hope we can make it all the more manageable by dispelling myths and offering detailed descriptions about some of the complex issues around modern bowel cancer surgery.

Operations for bowel cancer vary from relatively minor procedures, sometimes performed without hospital admission, to major operations taxing the technical expertise of the surgeon to its limits. Before looking at today's surgery, we think it would be useful to give a little of the background to its development.

The history of bowel cancer surgery

Before 1900, bowel cancer was less common and treatment was rather basic. In the late 1700s surgeons began making an 'artificial anus' or **colostomy** – an opening on the abdomen to allow faeces to escape – in some patients suffering from obstruction of the bowel due to cancer. At this time, this was a highly dangerous exercise, aimed at relieving dire symptoms, with no prospect of cure. In the early 1800s some surgeons resorted to pulling cancer tissue out through the anus to try to relieve patients afflicted by obstructing rectal cancers. Open abdominal surgery to deal with colon cancer (even if it could be diagnosed) was not even on the radar, as opening the abdomen was too dangerous to contemplate. By the late 1800s the lower part of the rectum was sometimes removed, leaving a gaping hole in the patient's bottom through which faeces would escape without control. Perhaps no surprise that this sort of surgery was not universally well regarded – surgeon Henry Smith commented on it thus in 1870:

> *Some surgeons a few years since were in the habit of performing excision of the lower part of the rectum when affected by cancer, but this proceeding must be looked upon as both barbarous and unscientific, and is now happily exploded from the catalogue of surgical operations.*

In fact it continued to be used and developed. A colostomy placed in the left lower part of the abdomen was added, which must have made it a little more tolerable for the recipients. Then, in

colostomy
Artificial opening of the colon onto the surface of the abdomen to allow faeces to leave the body, to be collected in a bag attached to the skin around the opening.

1908, the London surgeon, Ernest Miles, described his operation for rectal cancer which is still used for some patients today. Miles's operation differed from the procedure described above in that the surgeon opened the abdomen, a considerable undertaking at that time, to begin removing the rectum and to make a colostomy. Then he turned the patient on their side and completed the operation by cutting around the anus and upwards into the pelvis as described above, allowing the rectum and the cancer within it to be removed from below. The big difference between this and the earlier procedure was that it allowed the surgeon better access to the cancer by risking opening the abdomen, so that he could attempt a **radical** (i.e. potentially curative) excision. Cure, said Miles, was possible for the first time − but at considerable cost: − 40 per cent of Miles's patients died at, or soon after, the operation. It would be another 30 years before general surgical care of the surgical patient had improved enough to bring this dreadful death rate down to vaguely tolerable levels.

> **radical cancer surgery**
> Surgery aimed at cure, requiring removal of the primary tumour and its draining lymph glands.

Towards less extensive operations

In the 1920s pathologists examining the surgical specimens gradually became aware of something that was to lead to an important change in surgery by which a colostomy could be avoided. They found that the lymphatic drainage of the rectum (through which cancer cells sometimes spread to other parts of the body) was almost exclusively upwards, away from the anus. This meant that the lower part of the rectum and the anal muscles did not necessarily have to be removed to clear the tumour from the body.

The bowel ends, therefore, could be rejoined, thereby avoiding a colostomy. The idea that rectal cancer could be cured without making a colostomy was regarded by many surgeons as dangerous heresy in the late 1930s and 1940s, but gradually it became accepted. The gradual development of surgical technique meant that more and more patients could undergo **sphincter-saving surgery** and today, around 50 to 75 per cent of rectal cancer patients can undergo surgery that leaves their sphincters intact.

Technical developments from 1950 onwards

Telescope magic

An important step forward in the 1950s and 1960s was the coming of **fibreoptic** technology, whereby thousands of minute glass fibres could be held together in a bundle, each transmitting faithfully along its length the light that it picked up at its other end. Using this advance, long flexible **endoscopes** were developed that could transmit a picture, no matter what twists and turns were imposed along its length. Today the fibre bundle has been replaced by much higher resolution optical and camera technology.

These instruments can be inserted through any orifice to allow a view of the inside. For the large bowel the instrument is the colonoscope. Any disease process, including cancer and adenomas, can be seen with great clarity, and biopsies can be taken using long wire forceps. In some cases small tumours can actually be removed via the scope: a wire loop is passed down the scope, which can be placed around the tumour, after

---

sphincter-saving surgery

Radical rectal cancer surgery in which the bowel ends are re-joined after removal of the cancer, allowing preservation of the anal sphincters, so that faeces can be passed through the bottom as normal.

fibreoptics

Very clever technology in which thousands of long glass fibres are used to transmit a picture along their length; allowed the first examination of the inside of the colon, leading to a revolution in diagnosis and treatment of bowel diseases.

endoscope

endo- from the Greek *endos*, meaning 'within': hence an endoscope is an instrument used in the examination of the inside of the body.

which an electric current is passed through the loop, cutting off the tumour. Today quite complex procedures can be performed to remove extensive premalignant adenomas that previously would have required major surgery. All this can be done on the unanaesthetized patient without admitting them to the wards.

Surgical stapling

It's not only pieces of paper that can be stapled together. Using similar technology, much refined, pieces of bowel can be joined with great precision by **staple guns** that fire hundreds of minute titanium staples.

This advance has played a big part in extending the proportion of rectal cancer patients treated without a permanent colostomy by allowing safer **anastomosis** (joining of two pieces of bowel) in the most difficult area for access – deep in the pelvis.

Laparoscopic surgery

Technology continues ever forward. Now **laparoscopic surgery** can be performed through a small opening without conventional large abdominal incisions (so-called 'keyhole surgery').

Q This keyhole surgery sounds brilliant. Why don't all patients get it?

A Any new technology takes a long time to test, and then even longer to train all surgeons. We are only just reaching the point where it is accepted as being as good at curing patients as 'open' surgery, and as yet a minority of surgeons can do it. But watch – within a decade it will be as widely used as surgical stapling.

staple gun
Colloquial name for the family of medical instruments that allow minute metal staples to be used to join body tissues together, usually tubes, including bowel and arteries.

Q It sounds a bit rough to staple the bowel together. Is it?

A No, it's really not. The staples are very small, and there are very many of them, in two circles placed very close together. This method is reliable and quick, and now very widely used.

anastomosis
From the Greek meaning 'the making of a new opening' – in surgery it means joining two tubes (bowel, artery, ureters, etc.) together to restore a passage.

laparoscopic surgery
'Lapar-' from the Greek *laparos* meaning 'flank', but used in anatomy to mean the abdomen. Hence, surgery using an endoscope to view the inside of the abdomen without a large incision. Popularly known as 'keyhole surgery'.

After inflating the peritoneal cavity with gas, a telescope and several instruments can be inserted via 1–2 cm incisions, allowing full-scale surgery to remove the cancerous bowel and to rejoin the ends. As the technology develops and as surgeons gain the necessary skill and experience, it may well be that much of the surgery to be discussed below will be performed this way, with the promise of more comfortable and rapid postoperative recovery.

Surgical management today

Today the surgeon has a wide range of techniques and tools available to deal with the many different situations that may prevail. As discussed earlier, patients may present electively (allowing orderly assessment and discussion prior to treatment) or as an emergency. Management in these two categories differs substantially, so they will be discussed separately.

Elective surgery

Radical cancer surgery

The term 'radical' when applied to cancer surgery means that the operation is performed to achieve complete removal of a tumour so as to offer a chance of cure. In 1896 the American surgeon, Halsted, described the three principles of radical cancer surgery, namely, to remove:

✧ the primary tumour
✧ the lymphatic drainage tissue associated with it
✧ a margin of normal tissue around the tumour and lymphatic tissue, sufficient to ensure the best chance that all tumour cells have been removed.

myth
If you have surgery for bowel cancer, you are bound to wake up with a colostomy bag – for life.

fact
Simply not true today. It was never true for colon cancer and has not been true for rectal cancer for more than 50 years. Today around 85 per cent of rectal cancer patients will not need a permanent colostomy.

elective surgery
Surgery in which the time and place are 'elected', i.e. performed under optimum circumstances, as opposed to emergency surgery.

If a tumour is found not to be curable during investigation or at surgery, the overriding aim then is to do whatever can be done to keep the patient comfortable. Any such treatment is described as **palliative**. Surgery in this context will be discussed specifically in a later section.

palliative
From the Latin *palliare*, meaning literally 'to cover'. Medically it means to alleviate symptoms and suffering.

Preparation for surgery

These days measures are taken that make the length of hospital admission for major surgery ever shorter. One step is 'pre-assessment', in which the pre-operative examination and testing is done a week before admission. The patient comes to the outpatient department, mainly so that the surgeon can:

♦ check their general health and fitness for receiving an anaesthetic and major surgery, carry out routine blood tests and heart and lung tests if necessary

♦ ensure that the patient is clear on what is planned so that they can sign the surgery consent form.

The patient is usually admitted the day before surgery though there are moves towards coming in on the morning of the operation. On admission the anaesthetist will come along to check all the information about the patient's fitness for surgery.

Bowel preparation

Most surgeons prefer that the bowel is cleared out prior to surgery, perhaps making it easier to handle at operation, and perhaps making surgery safer, though many surgeons do not feel this is necessary. If 'bowel prep' is to be used, there are several available methods including:

oral laxatives

Medication to get the bowels working, either returning to normal in constipation, or overtime in bowel preparation. 'Oral' laxatives are taken by mouth.

irrigation

Used here euphemistically to indicate washing the bowel through by fluids instilled into the stomach via a tube.

nasogastric tube

Narrow plastic tube passed through the nose and down into the stomach through which medication or food can be injected or stomach contents removed.

stoma care nurse

A nurse specializing in training patients with, or about to have, a stoma.

stoma

From the Greek for 'mouth', in medicine it refers to an artificial opening onto the surface of the body, in this context a surgically constructed bowel opening.

✧ **oral laxatives** – the patient takes one or two doses of a strong laxative 24 hours before operation, leading to frequent visits to the lavatory for several hours

✧ **irrigation** – a small plastic tube is passed via the nostril into the stomach (**nasogastric tube**), followed by the drip feed of several litres of purgative solution that encourages the bowel to empty. Some patients find this method rather taxing, though it certainly works very well.

Meeting the stoma care nurse

Many hospitals have a specialist **stoma care nurse**, whose task is to help patients preparing for, or learning to live with a **stoma** – whether a colostomy or ileostomy (stomas using the colon and ileum [small bowel] respectively), whether it be temporary or permanent. If a stoma is likely, this nurse will visit before the operation. They will discuss the practicalities and choose the best site for the opening if it is needed. They will show the patient the sort of appliance to be used, and may stick it onto the skin so that they have some idea how it will feel.

myth
Nurses seem to be taking over. Surely doctors are the ones to make all the important decisions and nurses should just do what is ordered by the doctors.

fact
Nurses are certainly playing a bigger part by the year – and a jolly good thing too. The holistic approach (caring for the mind as well as the body) has always been central in nursing care, and this carries on into the more complex roles played by nurse specialists today. Frankly, nurses are often better in some tasks than junior doctors – and often times better than consultants!

Preventing blood clots

As with all major surgery there is a risk of blood clots forming in the leg veins (**deep vein thrombosis, DVT**), with a small but definite risk that these might break free and travel in the bloodstream to the lungs, where they can, if large enough, block the circulation (**pulmonary embolism**) causing severe acute illness or even death. However, this risk can be minimized, and many surgeons prescribe regular small doses of heparin to make the blood less ready to clot. This is given by injection under the skin of the abdomen or thigh. Another way to decrease the risk of clotting is the use of elasticated stockings which speed up the flow of blood in the leg veins.

Discussion of surgery

The consultant and their team will visit to try to answer any remaining questions. One thing the surgeon cannot do at this stage is to give a very clear prognosis, although the pre-operative scans give a fair idea. The most detailed prognosis possible has to await the pathology report on the tissue removed at the operation. The surgeon will talk through possible complications, so while remembering that the risks of surgery are generally fairly low, it is worth looking in a little detail at what the surgeon may discuss.

deep vein thrombosis (DVT)
Formation of blood clots in the veins deep within the calves. This happens due to trauma to the veins from pressure on the operating table, spontaneous increase in tendency of blood to clot during surgery, and slowed blood flow.

pulmonary embolism
Serious condition in which a blood clot becomes lodged in blood vessels in the lungs, partially or completely obstructing blood flow from the heart to the lungs, with a major risk of death.

my experience

I had a long discussion with my surgeon in outpatients before I was admitted for surgery but on the day I came into the ward I was a bag of nerves, and had forgotten all I had been told. Thank goodness my clinical nurse specialist was there to help me, and to make sure I asked all the last minute questions when the surgeon came round to see everybody who was on the operating list the next day. It is so important to make best use of that chance to talk before you hand yourself over to the surgical team.

Complications

There are both general complications – that can occur after any major operation – and those related directly to bowel surgery.

General complications

All major surgery carries a risk of problems to do with the circulation (heart attack, stroke), the lungs (chest infection, blood clot), the urinary system (infection or difficulty with emptying the bladder), and the operation wound (infection). These are kept to a minimum by careful pre-operative assessment for risk factors, and active attempts to prevent them by such measures as physiotherapy. If the patient is a smoker they will be encouraged to stop, as even a short break before the operation helps the lungs and airways to recover. Obesity is an important risk factor for all the complications listed above.

Special complications

Anastomotic leakage

A minor degree of leakage from an anastomosis is fairly common and non-threatening but in a few cases it is potentially very dangerous. Most anastomoses heal uneventfully despite faeces passing through the operated bowel within a few days. If at the end of the operation the surgeon feels that the anastomosis is at more than usual risk of leaking, they will make a temporary **ileostomy** 'upstream' to prevent faeces travelling through the sutured (surgical word for 'stitched') bowel while it heals. Sometimes,

ileostomy
Opening made in the small bowel (ileum) to allow it to drain into a bag on the abdominal surface.

however, an anastomosis which did not seem to be at particular risk, and was therefore not protected by an ileostomy will, nevertheless, spring a leak. If so the patient may develop a temperature, perhaps some abdominal pain and the bowel may become sluggish, causing nausea, decreased bowel movements and distension of the abdomen.

The body's defences may deal with this sort of leak by wrapping protective tissue around the affected area, preventing the escaped faeces from causing serious infection. Sometimes the situation is more serious, with leakage of faeces throughout the abdominal cavity (causing peritonitis) or out to the surface through the surgical wound, or both. This may require further surgery to clean up and to make the bowel safe, sometimes by taking the anastomosis apart and bringing out a colostomy, or by making a temporary ileostomy or colostomy. The patient may then need a spell in the intensive care unit until the crisis has passed. Some months later the stoma will be closed if all is well.

Nerve damage

Nerves supplying the bladder and controlling sexual function lie close to the rectum and so risk being damaged during difficult rectal cancer surgery. This may show itself with:

✧ the patient not being able to pass urine spontaneously (**neuropathic bladder**). This will become apparent on removal of the bladder **catheter**, placed at the time of surgery. The catheter will be re-inserted to see if the bladder has recovered spontaneously a day or two later, perhaps

neuropathic bladder
Bladder that has lost its ability to contract and squeeze out urine, due to nerve damage during surgery, or sometimes due to radiotherapy.

catheter
A soft rubber tube placed in the bladder at the beginning of the operation to drain urine into a bag during and immediately after the operation.

with the help of medication. If this does not work out, a urologist may come to test bladder function, perhaps prescribe further medication, or suggest the patient keep their catheter for some weeks (hoping that normal function will resume), or perform a small operation to restore urinary flow

✧ male patients, following discharge from hospital, experiencing impotence and/or sterility (it seems that women do not usually develop an equivalent sexual failure). 'Impotence' means failure of erection, while 'sterility' is due to failure of ejaculation. The risk is greater in total rectal excision. Post-operative anxiety can also cause impotence. These problems, whatever the cause, are often helped with prescription medicines, of which sildenafil (Viagra) is one of several options.

What happens on operation day?

About one hour before the operation, the patient gets their pre-operative medication – the 'pre-med' – an injection in the buttock or leg, making the patient sleepily at ease, and drying the mouth and air passages, making anaesthesia safer. A ward nurse accompanies the patient to theatre.

The anaesthetic room

The patient goes off to sleep after an injection in the back of the hand; the injection also paralyzes all the muscles, making it possible for the anaesthetist to insert a breathing tube, called the endotracheal tube. This is a plastic tube passed through the mouth and into the windpipe (trachea). It is held in place by a soft balloon in the trachea and allows the anaesthetist complete control of breathing during surgery. (Paralysis also makes it much easier for the surgeon to operate.)

Then the anaesthetist sets up a 'drip' in the arm to give fluids and blood during the operation, and a urine drainage tube ('catheter') is usually inserted. They may also put lines into an artery and a vein to check blood pressure and the efficiency of the circulation. Finally the anaesthetist may put a small tube into the spinal canal ('epidural catheter') through which to deliver painkillers. This is extremely useful both during the operation and for several days after. All this is a far cry from what the anaesthetist could contribute even just a generation ago. Now the patient is taken into the operating theatre.

The operation

Which operation type is selected depends on the site of the tumour, but whatever the operation it has three main elements:

✧ inspection of everything inside the abdomen
✧ removal of the part of the bowel containing the tumour
✧ rejoining (anastomosis) of the bowel or the formation of a colostomy.

These three elements will be dealt with separately.

Initial inspection

The abdomen is opened vertically down the middle (unless laparoscopy is used, as described elsewhere). The surgeon carefully checks the primary tumour, the rest of the bowel, and looks for distant spread.

Now the surgeon can decide how best to proceed. These days, with such accurate pre-operative tests, it is unusual for the surgeon to need to change tack, but sometimes unexpected findings change the operative plan.

Getting the cancer out

resection
Surgical term for the complete or partial removal of a body organ.

If radical **resection** is to proceed, the next phase is removal of the primary tumour, including its lymphatic drainage and a margin of normal tissue. If it has invaded surrounding structures, the surgeon should already know from the scans. It will probably have been worked out before the operation that an extended resection is likely, and an appropriate team will have been lined up, perhaps including a urologist, gynaecologist, orthopaedic or plastic surgeons (or any combination thereof!).

As operations of the colon and rectum are now described, it would be worth checking back to the descriptions of bowel anatomy given in Chapter 1. The techniques for removing colon and rectal cancer differ.

Colon cancer

colectomy
Operation to remove a part (hemicolectomy) or all (total colectomy) of the colon.

The operation to remove a colonic tumour is called a **colectomy**; if the tumour is in the right (or left) colon the operation is a right (or left) hemi ('half') colectomy (see Figures 7.1 and 7.2). Then there are transverse and sigmoid colectomies. Often 30–40 cm of bowel is removed to ensure that all the associated lymph

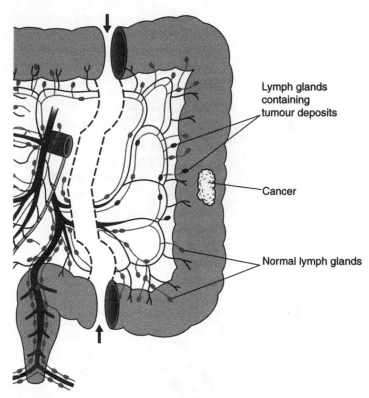

Lymph glands
containing
tumour deposits

Cancer

Normal lymph glands

Figure 7.1 Left hemicolectomy. The arrows and dotted lines indicate the line along which the surgeon cuts away the segment of bowel and the lymph glands and arteries connected with it. Such wide removal is necessary to clear away any lymph glands that might contain tumour.

glands are taken but, perhaps surprisingly, this has little if any effect on bowel function afterwards.

The surgeon begins by freeing the segment from surrounding structures to make it more accessible. Then the mesentery is cut away from the back of the abdominal cavity; the main arteries and veins within it are cut and tied at their

anterior resection
Original name for sphincter-saving rectal resection. First described in the 1930s, and so named to differentiate it from the old, non-radical operation in which the rectum was removed from below and behind, without significant incursion into the abdomen ('posterior resection').

(a)

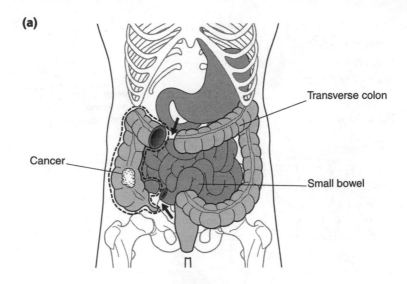

Transverse colon

Cancer

Small bowel

(b)

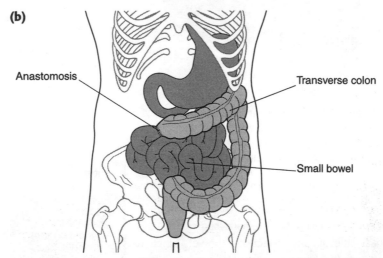

Anastomosis

Transverse colon

Small bowel

Figure 7.2 Right hemicolectomy. (a) shows the extent of resection; as in Fig 7.1, a wide clearance is necessary to maximize the chance of cure. (b) shows what happens after anastomosis (rejoining of the ends). The cut end of the small bowel has been stitched to the cut end of the transverse colon. The bowel resumes its normal function rapidly after surgery.

origin, taking all the lymph glands along them. Finally the bowel is cut across above and below the tumour and removed, and the removed tissue is sent to the pathologist.

Rectal cancer

It is commonly thought that rectal cancer surgery always means a permanent colostomy. True once, but today 85 per cent of patients do not need one. In the majority the bowel ends are rejoined, a procedure known as **anterior resection** (see key term box on p.107). If the whole rectum must be removed, the operation is **abdomino-perineal excision**. Let us look at these operations in more detail.

Abdomino-perineal excision of the rectum (APER)

Sometimes known as Miles's operation after the surgeon who devised it, this operation was first performed a century ago. It consists of the radical removal of the whole rectum and anal canal and the formation of a colostomy in the left lower part of the abdominal wall (see Figure 7.3).

Q Is it really true that only specialist bowel surgeons should carry out rectal cancer surgery?

A Difficult one. Most bowel surgeons think so, and this is happening more and more. Colon cancer surgery is less complex, so that general surgeons may deal with these cases, particularly if they are admitted as emergencies; but nevertheless we are moving towards bowel surgeons doing it all, leaving other surgeons to concentrate on what they do best.

Q How come an operation invented 100 years ago (APER) is still used today? Surely things have moved on.

A Yes, they have, but in around 15 per cent of rectal cancer cases this is still the best operation. Today the surgery is done better, patients are chosen very carefully using modern investigations, and pre-operative therapy is used more – hence the growing success of this and other rectal cancer surgery.

abdomino-perineal excision of therectum(APER)
The original radical operation for rectal cancer. Today two surgeons, working from the abdomen and perineum (area around anus and scrotum or vulva), jointly excise the rectum.

(a)

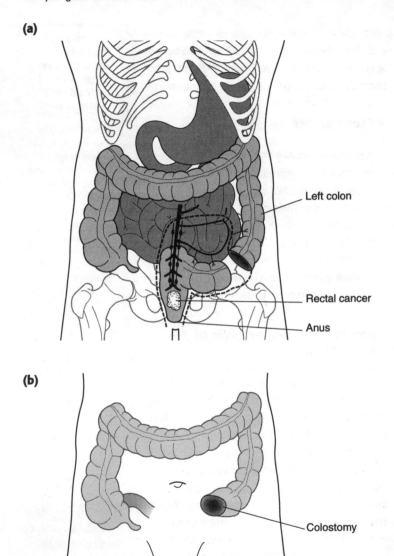

Left colon

Rectal cancer

Anus

(b)

Colostomy

Figure 7.3 Abdomino-perineal excision of the rectum.
(a) shows the extent of resection – in this operation the
whole rectum and part of the colon are removed, with
the inferior mesenteric artery and associated lymph
glands. (b) shows the final result – the cut end of the
colon is brought to the surface to form a colostomy.

The patient lies on their back on the table with their legs suspended up and apart, allowing one surgeon to work on the abdominal end and a second surgeon to operate via the perineum (the area around and in front of the anus). At the outset the second surgeon closes the anus with a stitch to prevent faeces contaminating the operation.

The abdominal part of the operation begins with the **mobilization** of the sigmoid colon and upper rectum. The major artery and vein supplying the rectum are cut across close to the aorta (the body's main artery), thereby ensuring that all lymph glands around them are removed. The bowel is cut across in the upper part of the sigmoid colon. Great care is taken to preserve the nerves supplying the bladder and organs of sexual function, some of which pass downwards into the pelvis behind the rectum. The operation then proceeds downwards into the pelvis, aiming to remove with great care all of the tissues to the sides of and behind the rectum (known as the **mesorectum**, containing the blood vessels and lymphatics serving the rectum). This dissection is crucial to the success of the operation and has been called **total mesorectal excision (TME)**. The surgeon must work in what has been called the 'holy plane' (see Figures 7.4 and 7.5) to ensure the precise removal of the mesorectum and its contents. The vagina in women or the bladder and seminal vesicles (the two small bags at the base of the bladder where semen is stored) in men must be separated from the front of the rectum. The dissection is carried deeply into the pelvis, to link up with that of the perineal surgeon.

mobilization
Surgical dissection to free a structure from surrounding tissues.

mesorectum
Bundle of fatty and fibrous tissue wrapped around the rectum, mainly at the back, and containing the blood vessels, and very importantly the lymph glands draining the rectum.

total mesorectal excision (TME)
Name given to a meticulous surgical dissection of the rectum and mesorectum, aimed at removing them with great care to avoid splitting the mesorectum and potentially exposing the tumour that might have spread into it. Technique emphasized by one of the leading rectal cancer surgeons of the twentieth century, Professor Bill Heald, in contrast to widely used 'blunt dissection' in which the rectum was more or less pulled out of the pelvis.

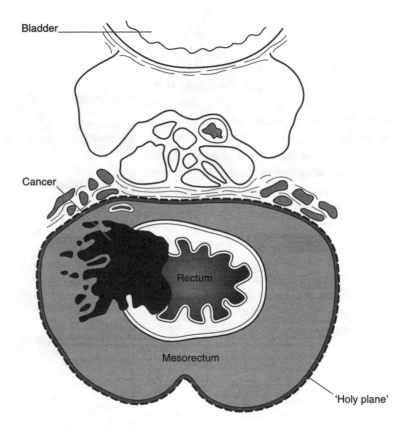

Figure 7.4 Horizontal view of mesorectal dissection in the 'holy plane'. The surgeon dissects around the mesorectum with care, as any incursion inside the holy plane risks exposing the cancer or leaving involved lymph glands behind.

pelvic floor
Funnel-shaped sheet of muscle, known to anatomists as *levator ani*, that is spread across the bottom of the pelvis as a diaphragm, through which the rectum, vagina and urethra pass to reach 'the outside'.

Meanwhile the perineal surgeon will have begun by cutting around the anus to reach the lower surface of the **pelvic floor**. This is a thin sheet of muscle attached to the bony sides of the pelvis sweeping downwards to surround the anorectal junction (the point where the rectum joins the anal canal). The pelvic floor is intimately

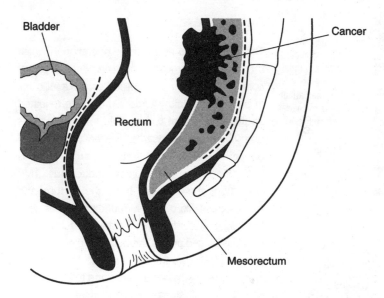

Figure 7.5 Side view of mesorectal dissection in the 'holy plane' (dotted lines). Again, care must be taken when dissecting around the mesorectum.

wrapped around any tumour in the lowest part of the rectum, so it should be left undisturbed as the perineal surgeon separates it to pass upwards to meet the approach of the abdominal surgeon. Once the rectum and surrounding tissues have been dissected free, the specimen is removed through the perineal wound.

The wounds are closed and a colostomy made. A tube is usually placed in the pelvis, coming out through the abdominal wall, to remove any blood or tissue fluid that may collect.

Q What if I <u>really</u> <u>can't</u> face having a colostomy?

A Surgeons must take the patient's feelings and fears fully into account when advising on surgery. Sometimes the surgeon will feel that a 'join-up' operation is possible but is less likely to cure, or more likely to result in poor function afterwards.

A At other times the surgeon may know that cure is simply not possible without a colostomy. They must tell the patient all there is to know, and ultimately the patient has to make up their mind, sometimes just having to accept the inevitable.

en bloc **removal**
Cancer surgery in which the organ of origin of the cancer and surrounding organ(s) that have been invaded by the cancer are taken in one 'block' to avoid exposing the cancer and shedding malignant cells.

ileal conduit
A simple bladder replacement, in which a 15 cm piece of bowel, usually ileum, is dissected free but retaining its blood supply. The ureters are stitched to one end, while the other is brought to the skin surface as a stoma.

urostomy
The outer end of an ileal conduit.

Anterior resection

This is the name given to the operation in which the surgeon removes the segment of bowel containing the tumour, but leaves the anal canal in place; the healthy ends can then be re-joined so that the patient will be able to pass motions normally again afterwards. The early part of the operation – rectal mobilization – is the same as that used in APER. Using meticulous TME dissection, the surgeon frees the rectum and mesorectum from the surrounding tissues to a level several centimetres below the tumour. A clamp is placed across the bowel and an assistant passes a tube into the lower part of the rectum to wash out any remaining faeces and to kill any free cancer cells. A stapler is used to seal the lower rectum before the piece of bowel containing the tumour is removed, leaving behind the lower end ready for the final phase, the rejoining of the bowel (see Figure 7.6).

En bloc removal of advanced tumours

It is usually fairly clear from pre-operative scans whether any surrounding organs – vagina, uterus, bladder, prostate gland, sacrum or small bowel – have been invaded. Most of these parts can be cut out if necessary, but if the bladder has to be completely removed, a new way out for urine has to be made. This involves the construction of an **ileal conduit** – an artificial bladder made from a short segment of small bowel. The cut ends of the ureters are sutured to one end of the conduit while the other end is brought to the surface of the abdomen as a stoma (**urostomy**), so that urine can drain freely into a plastic bag appliance.

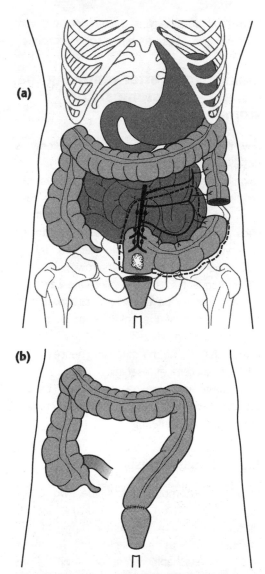

Figure 7.6 Anterior resection of the rectum. (a) The extent of resection. This is the procedure if the tumour can be removed safely without taking the lowest part of the rectum and anus. (b) After anastomosis. The cut end of the colon is joined to the 'rectal stump'. This is sometimes very difficult if the pelvis is narrow (most often in stocky men).

This sort of surgery is uncommon and very challenging; it is best done in a specialist centre.

Making good after removing the tumour – anastomosis or stoma?

Now the surgeon must restore the anatomy as closely as possible to normal. If a segment of colon or rectum has been removed, the ends can be joined; if, however, the rectum and anus have been removed, a colostomy is necessary. If the ends are to be joined, the loss of the storage (reservoir) function of the rectum by its replacement with relatively narrow colon, can lead to frequent visits to the toilet. One way to get around this may be to make a **colopouch**, in which the end of the colon is doubled over, opened and then stitched to produce a tube that is wider than the normal colon and hence may be a better replacement reservoir.

> **colopouch**
> A surgical manoeuvre to try to turn narrow colon into a replacement for the more capacious rectum.

An anastomosis can be made either using a stapling instrument or by the time-honoured method of 'hand-suturing'.

Stapled anastomosis

Stapled anastomosis unites the two bowel ends – the colon and rectum – by the placement of two concentric rings of fine titanium staples using a staple 'gun'. To achieve this, the detachable head, or 'anvil', of the instrument is stitched into the colon. The 'barrel' of the staple gun is then inserted through the anus. A metal spike is deployed from its tip, passing through the upper end of the previously divided rectum; the spike is then attached to the anvil. By turning a screw in the handle of the gun, outside the anus, the colon and rectum are brought tightly together, the gun is fired by pulling a lever, the staples are deployed and the bowel ends are joined. It is then possible to remove the gun, with the anvil attached to it, via the anus.

Hand-sutured anastomosis

This isn't used as much now except in cases where the cancer was at the top of the rectum, or if there is some technical problem preventing the use of the staple gun. One or two rings of sutures are placed by hand, achieving the same result as with stapling.

There is a variant of the hand-sutured anastomosis known as **coloanal anastomosis**, by which the bowel ends are joined via a short telescope passed into the anus. This is used if the whole rectum has been removed down to its junction with the anal canal. Having removed the cancer, and with the surgeon seated facing the perineum (the patient's legs held apart on stirrups), the assistant delivers the cut end of the colon down through the pelvis to the anus. Using a small instrument to hold the anus open the surgeon then sutures the end of the colon to the middle of the anal canal.

The surgeon may put the bowel anastomosis temporarily 'out of circuit' by making an upstream stoma, which can be closed a couple of months later when the anastomosis has healed soundly. Most surgeons routinely make such a stoma when the join is very low, particularly with coloanal anastomosis.

> **coloanal anastomosis**
> The very lowest possible sphincter-saving procedure, in which, after resection of the entire rectum, the colon – either a simple end or a colopouch – is sutured into the anal canal.

Laparoscopic (keyhole) surgery

This type of surgery started with the gynaecologists and has spread gradually to other surgical specialties. It has a well established place in surgery of the gall bladder and stomach, and in some types of hernia. More latterly it has come to bowel surgery; it presents great technical challenges due to the relative complexity of bowel anatomy. Potentially any operation for bowel cancer – except in procedures for advanced or recurrent cancers – might be performed this way.

Initially the surgeon distends the abdomen with gas to provide a space within which to manoeuvre instruments. Then a small opening is made below the umbilicus (belly button) to allow insertion of a telescope, through which the surgeon can see what he is doing – this is controlled by an assistant throughout the operation. The operator and the team view their progress on monitors placed opposite them (see Figure 7.7). Several 'ports' are placed in the abdominal wall; these are plastic devices through which dissecting, manipulating and suturing instruments can be inserted to perform the operation. Great skill is required to do the same sort of dissection performed in conventional operations, but with one enormous difference: it is vital to maintain scrupulous **haemostasis**, that is, there must be no bleeding, as this cannot be dealt with easily. Special instruments are therefore used to do the bloodless cutting, and they work incredibly effectively. After mobilization and resection are completed, a short incision is made to allow removal. If there is an anastomosis to be made, this can be done within the

haemostasis
The state of 'no bleeding'. Surgeons seek to achieve haemostasis at all times – sometimes easier said than done!

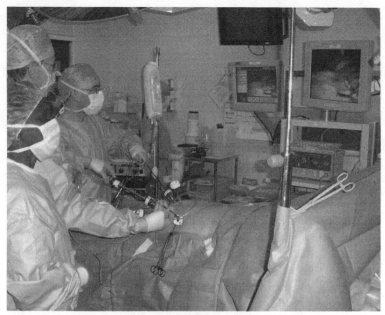

Figure 7.7 Laparoscopic surgery ('keyhole' surgery). After distending the abdomen with gas to allow a view of the internal organs, the surgeon has inserted a camera and several grasping and cutting instruments. By viewing the camera image on the monitors opposite them, the team can perform very delicate and precise surgery without having to make the conventional long incision in the abdomen.

abdomen, but this calls for the highest levels of dexterity. Often the surgeon will bring the cut ends out through the hole made to bring out the cancer specimen, join the ends in conventional fashion, and return it to the abdomen. Sometimes the surgeon may find that he cannot continue to make progress laparoscopically, and has to 'convert', that is, to open the abdomen with a larger incision to finish the operation. Generally, the more experienced the surgeon, the fewer cases are converted.

The keyhole approach has been shown to cause less abdominal discomfort and therefore quicker recuperation. Trials suggest it is just as effective in treating cancer as open surgery. We will see how the field evolves.

Other types of surgery

Surgery for liver metastases

Although liver metastases are generally a sign that cure is not possible, sometimes they can be dealt with surgically, giving the patient some chance if all visible tumour can be removed, with about a 30 per cent prospect of cure.

If the metastases are potentially removable, it is usual to do this at a second operation, once the patient has recovered from the first. This allows further assessment of operability. Liver resection is a major undertaking, and should generally performed by a specialist surgeon.

Surgery for locally recurrent cancer

A minority of patients who develop local recurrence in the months or years following surgery are suitable for an attempt at surgical cure. If symptoms or routine post-operative tests lead to this diagnosis, a string of tests must be performed to answer these important questions:

- ✧ Is the abnormality seen on the scan truly a recurrence, or might it be something else, such as scarring from previous surgery or inflammation from an anastomotic leak?
- ✧ Is this a single area of recurrence, or is there disease elsewhere that would make cure impossible?

✧ Does the recurrence involve any structure that might not allow the cancer to be removed completely?

✧ Is the patient fit enough and willing to undergo major and potentially debilitating surgery?

If the answers to all these questions are favourable, then serious consideration can be given to surgery. As with locally advanced primary surgery, this is usually a matter for a team of experts, and the surgery is much as was discussed earlier in that context.

Non-radical surgery

Occasionally a cancer is small enough to be treated by a 'non-radical' operation – one that removes only the primary tumour and does not remove the lymph glands. This may be done by:

✧ local excision
✧ colonoscopic excision.

non-radical surgery
Any operation for cancer that does not fulfil Halstead's three conditions for radical surgery; usually indicates that the primary tumour has been removed but the lymph drainage left in place.

Local excision

This can be done if the patient has a small cancer (up to three or four centimetres across) in the lower rectum. The risk of local recurrence is higher and the certainty of cure less than for radical surgery, but against this must be reckoned the lesser risk of major complications and even of death due to the surgery itself. This approach is particularly suited to the frail and elderly. Only around five per cent of rectal cancers are appropriate for local excision, though this may increase if more early tumours are detected by screening.

Local excision is performed with the patient in either the 'lithotomy' position (on their back with the legs held fully flexed in stirrups) or in the 'jackknife' position (on their front with the operating table bent in the middle, at the level of the perineum, with the legs bent downwards in an upside down V-shape allowing access to the anus), depending on the site of the tumour. The surgeon places an instrument in the anus to hold it widely open. After injecting adrenaline solution to minimize bleeding, a disc of bowel wall is removed including the tumour and a one centimetre cuff of normal tissue around it. The hole produced can then be sutured. Another technique, **transanal endoscopic microsurgery (TEM)** is used for tumours higher in the rectum. A very fancy telescope is inserted through the anus, through which the surgeon has a stereoscopic view; instruments can be inserted through the scope to remove the tumour and to mend the hole.

A few days later the pathologist tells the surgeon whether their examination is favourable. If he thinks otherwise the surgeon will have to discuss a conventional radical operation with the patient to ensure the best chance of cure.

> **transanal endoscopic microsurgery (TEM)**
> Technique using a large calibre endoscope that allows precise excision of rectal tumours under stereoscopic vision.

Colonoscopic excision

The colonoscope is an extremely useful tool for some early-stage bowel cancers. The colonoscope can be used to locate and remove a malignant polyp by lassooing it with a wire loop that can be tightened so that the polyp is cut off using an electric current. This is a straightforward procedure from the patient's point of view, carried out under mild sedation and usually as an outpatient. It can only be performed for this particularly favourable, and less common, type of early cancer. It can also be used to remove benign adenomas, small or large. Before the colonoscope was invented, open abdominal surgery was necessary to treat these conditions.

Emergency surgery

Around 30 per cent of patients with bowel cancer come to hospital only after developing complications of the disease, **obstruction** or **perforation**. Of this group three quarters arrive with obstruction, the rest with perforation and peritonitis. Both situations are life-threatening.

Resuscitation and preparation for surgery

The obstructed bowel becomes loaded with large volumes of fluid, deriving originally from the blood circulation. This reduces the blood volume, which may make the patient very ill. Peritonitis induces a state of shock due to the inflammation and infection in the abdomen and the bloodstream. Rapid assessment and treatment are vital. Patients are often unfit due to other health problems and these will need sorting out as well. Unfortunately such patients often do not get to hospital until the evening or night; in cases of obstruction, rather than rushing to theatre there and then, it is usual to spend more time resuscitating the patient, and saving surgery till the daylight hours, when a more senior and rested surgical team will be around and the patient will have been made fitter by resuscitation. In peritonitis, however, once resuscitation has been completed, surgery should be performed straightaway, whatever the hour.

obstruction
Complete blockage of the intestine, causing sudden severe illness. The bowel upstream becomes distended, the bowel does not empty, vomiting may occur, and the patient has severe colicky abdominal pain.

perforation
The bowel has burst, leading to faecal contamination of the abdominal cavity and hence peritonitis.

resuscitation
In this context, refers to the process of treatment to replace lost fluid via an intravenous drip, injection of antibiotics if necessary, delivery of oxygen – all aimed at making the patient fitter for surgery.

dynamic stent
Wire mesh tube that can be passed through an obstructed bowel segment, which on deployment begins to widen its calibre in order to open up the tight area, so relieving the obstruction.

An important development in the management of intestinal obstruction is the **dynamic stent**. This is essentially a short tube of wire mesh. Either through a colonoscope or under X-ray guidance (or both) the stent is passed across the obstruction; on deployment, it expands, gently opening up the obstruction. The patient can then be operated electively a few days later, when their general state will have improved.

Aims of emergency surgery

The immediate aim is to save the patient's life: other considerations, including cure of the cancer, take second place for the moment. As with elective surgery, the emergency procedure has three phases:

◇ initial assessment
◇ treating the disease
◇ considering whether to perform an anastomosis or make a stoma.

Opening the abdomen and initial assessment

If the bowel is obstructed, special care is required as the tensely distended bowel can burst. If the bowel has perforated prior to operation, the surgeon's first task is to clean up by suction. Then the surgeon will try to prevent further leakage by gently clamping the bowel. Once under control thorough washing ('lavage') is performed.

As there will have been no pre-operative scan it is down to the surgeon to assess the state of the cancer; they must decide whether to remove it at this operation or to do the minimum to sort out the emergency and leave tackling the cancer for another day.

Tackling the tumour

Usually the surgeon will aim to resect, following the broad principles used in elective surgery, though this may be made more difficult if the bowel is obstructed. Occasionally the surgeon may simply make a colostomy upstream of the tumour to relieve obstruction or prevent further leakage from a perforation.

Anastomosis or stoma?

A surgeon will make an anastomosis if the situation is favourable, though often with a precautionary temporary stoma upstream. If anastomosis does not seem sensible, the upstream cut end of the colon is brought to the surface as a colostomy while the other end is closed and returned to the abdomen. This is known as **Hartmann's procedure**. If the patient recovers well, a later operation is performed to join the ends again.

Surgery in the incurable case

Sometimes the surgeon finds that the disease is beyond cure, either because the primary tumour cannot be separated from structures around it, or that it has spread via the bloodstream to other organs.

In the incurable patient the decision has to be made whether to remove the primary tumour; in many cases it may be better to rely on the beneficial effects of chemotherapy to slow the disease rather than subject the patient to the disruption of surgery. If obstruction is imminent, a stent can be used, as mentioned in the section on emergency surgery.

> ### Hartmann's procedure
> Old operation still used today in which a diseased area in the rectum or sigmoid colon is removed, the rectum closed off, and the end of the colon delivered to make a colostomy.

Stomas – colostomy and ileostomy

Stoma (a Greek word meaning 'mouth') is an artificial opening in the bowel. It may be called a 'colostomy' (a 'colon-stoma') or an 'ileostomy' (an 'ileum-stoma'). Many people today are still under the false impression that the treatment of bowel cancer always means 'having a bag'. This was once true for rectal cancer, but today it is grossly inaccurate (no more than 20 per cent of rectal cancer patients need a permanent colostomy), and it was never true for colon cancer.

Types of stoma

Temporary or permanent?

Stomas are made for two main reasons:

✧ as a stop-gap to protect a vulnerable anastomosis while it heals. In this situation a *temporary* stoma is made, usually an ileostomy
✧ as a permanent measure, to replace the function of the rectum and anus.

Colostomy or ileostomy?

While most patients who need a permanent stoma as part of the treatment of bowel cancer will have a colostomy, if the whole colon and rectum must be removed the ileum is the only part of the bowel available to make a permanent stoma. Temporary stomas are usually ileostomies.

Loop or terminal stoma?

Temporary stomas are made by bringing the bowel through the abdominal wall to the skin surface, opening the bowel and suturing it to the skin. This is known as a **loop stoma**. If the stoma is to be permanent, the cut end, or termination, of the bowel is brought to the skin surface, hence the name, **terminal colostomy**.

Where are stomas sited?

A stoma could be sited anywhere on the abdomen but, in general, whether temporary or permanent, a colostomy will be placed in the left lower abdomen (left iliac fossa) and an ileostomy in the right iliac fossa for ease of access and care.

Choosing the site

The stoma should be located on flat skin, away from bony prominences, scars, skin creases and the umbilicus. It should pass through the rectus abdominis muscle, which runs as a strip either side of the midline. The patient must be able to see it easily, sometimes very difficult if the patient is obese. It is almost impossible to gauge accurately where the stoma should be sited when the patient is asleep on the operating table, so it is very important to choose the spot pre-operatively. Having chosen a likely spot with the patient lying on the bed, it must be checked with the patient standing and sitting (skin creases due to rolls of fat can appear from nowhere!); only then should the chosen spot be marked with an indelible pen to guide the surgeon at the operation.

How is a stoma made?

Terminal stoma

A two to three centimetre circular opening ('trephine') in the abdominal wall, sited as

loop stoma
Usually using ileum, a temporary stoma in which the bowel is not cut across, but is brought to the abdominal surface, opened and sutured, producing an effective stoma that is easily closed at a later date when no longer needed.

terminal colostomy
Sounds ominous, but simply refers to a colostomy where the cut end (termination) of the colon is used to make the stoma.

outlined above, is made as the first step in the operation. This channel is then left alone while the operation proceeds. As the final step the cut end of the bowel is delivered through the trephine, the main abdominal incision is closed and the stoma is stitched to the skin. A colostomy is a very simple opening, almost flush with the skin; an ileostomy is constructed slightly differently – a small spout, two to three centimetres long, is made by drawing out twice that length of bowel and doubling it back on itself before suturing it to the skin. This ensures that the bowel content is delivered well down into the bag rather than at skin level as the effluent is very irritating to the skin. Having finished making the stoma, a plastic bag appliance is attached to the abdominal wall to enclose it, protecting the skin immediately around the stoma and ready to collect the effluent.

Loop stoma

Through a trephine made as described above, the loop of bowel is brought through it, and may be supported at skin level by a plastic or glass rod, which is taken out a week later. The bowel is opened and the cut edges stitched to the skin and a bag attached.

Post-operative recovery

These days elective surgery for bowel cancer is much safer, the great majority coming through without a hiccup. Nevertheless around one per cent of patients may die in the first month after the operation and rather more will suffer complications of varying seriousness. To keep things as safe as possible, the nursing and medical staff have a routine set of procedures which unsuspecting patients and their visitors may find baffling.

Tubes, drains, and bags

On return to the ward there will be several tubes or other appliances attached to the patient:

✧ An intravenous drip running via a tube attached to the arm or the side of the neck. Through this the patient will receive around three litres of fluid per 24 hours in place of the normal intake by mouth. If the patient needs blood this will be given via the drip, and it is also a convenient route for the administration of drugs, such as antibiotics.

✧ There may be an epidural catheter (explained on page 105) to deliver reliable pain control for the first few days.

✧ A nasogastric tube, passing through the nose and down into the stomach. This drains the digestive juices that are not required and which can cause nausea and even vomiting. However, many surgeons have found that this tube is not routinely necessary and have dispensed with it.

✧ The bladder will be emptying via a catheter which drains into a bag. This makes it possible to keep an eye on the volume of urine being produced, hence helping with fluid prescription; it also relieves the patient of the need to get out of bed to pass urine in the first few post-operative days.

✧ There may be drainage tubes to remove any fluid or blood which may collect, helping to prevent infections and leakage from the anastomosis. Drains usually stay in for around two to four days.

✧ As discussed above, there may be a stoma bag. The bowel will empty into the bag a few days after the operation; the nurses will look after it completely to start with, but as the patient recovers they will be trained in its care.

Medication

Infections, in particular in the wound, are kept to a minimum with antibiotics for a short period. The first dose is usually given at the beginning of the operation, with two more doses in the next 24 hours.

Pain relieving drugs (analgesics) will be required during recovery. Their obvious aim is to kill pain, and as a result they make breathing and movement easier, thereby helping to avoid chest and other complications. In the first few days analgesia may be given via an epidural catheter. A good alternative is PCA – patient controlled analgesia – whereby patients can give themselves small 'slugs' of morphine, or an equivalent, directly into a vein simply by pressing a button. A machine counts the doses and prevents over-dosing. This is a much better method than the rather outdated four hourly injection into the buttock or thigh! When the patient is able to drink, analgesia is taken by mouth.

Q My friend works in the hospital and knows about these things. She says there's a whole bunch of things I should never eat again after my operation. Is this really true?

A No, it's not. Once you feel up to it, you should try anything you like. If you find a food that upsets your tummy, you may want to avoid it. There is no need to go beyond the usual dos and don'ts of a healthy diet.

Diet

Food may be withheld for a few days; this does not matter for a short period, but as soon as the bowel shows signs of working, the patient will be offered small amounts of water and other drinks to start with, soon followed by progression to a light diet and then on to normal food several days after the operation. There are no particular dietary needs or restrictions after bowel cancer surgery, except for a few minor rules for some patients with a stoma (more on this later). Some surgeons offer their patients drink and food from the day of surgery as part of a potentially revolutionary change in post-operative care, known as **enhanced recovery programme (ERP)**. This has been developed in parallel with laparoscopic surgery and aims to shorten hospital stay through wider use of epidurals, immediate return to drinking and eating, rapid mobilization and minimal use of drains and tubes.

Discussion of outcome

When the patient has recovered sufficiently, the surgical team will discuss what has been done and what the future is likely to hold. If all has gone well the patient and relatives will be reassured at an early stage, usually within 24 hours or so of the operation. Full discussion must await the pathologist's report but patients and their families differ in the information that they seek. All need to know about speed of recovery and the effects of surgery on bowel activity, stomas, etc., but most important is the chance of cure.

The surgeon, once armed with the pathologist's report (usually about a week after the operation), will be able to tell the patient the **Dukes' stage** of the tumour, that is the pathological stage of advancement, and this will give a good idea of

enhanced recovery programme (ERP)
Increasingly popular post-operative regimen, which is aimed at getting the patient fitter quicker, leading to earlier discharge from hospital.

Dukes' staging system
Method for applying information gathered by the pathologist during examination of operative specimen to estimate the likelihood of cure. It also assists in deciding whether post-operative chemotherapy is advisable.

the percentage chance that the patient is cured. However, the surgeon may have evidence from the operation that the patient is not curable and obviously this information must be imparted with great care, usually after careful explanation and consultation with close relatives, who may play a central role in helping the patient to understand and deal with the information. They may feel that the patient should not be told the full story in these circumstances; the surgeon will certainly take these feelings fully into account though the patient's right to know must also always be remembered. The whole problem of imparting information and discussing its implications with patients and their families can be very complex sometimes. Despite the best intentions and efforts of the staff, however, patients and relatives may be confused by the barrage of technicalities directed at them; if this is the case, they should always feel free to ask to see the doctors again, including the consultant, to discuss things further. The cancer nurse specialist plays an invaluable role in supporting and explaining over the ensuing days.

Getting up and about

Lying motionless in bed after major surgery predisposes to complications – chest infection, blood clots and bed sores. An important part of post-operative care, therefore, is early encouragement to move. Initially this means breathing exercises and active leg movements in bed, but within a day or two the patient will be out of bed to take short walks, aided by the nurses. Sitting crumpled in a bedside chair is not a good alternative!

Care of the operation wound

Unless there is a stoma, the only part of the surgeon's handiwork visible to the patient is the skin wound. If all goes well the stitches or clips can be removed about ten days after the operation. This is a simple and, surprisingly for most, pain-free procedure; if the patient goes home before the tenth post-operative day, the sutures can be removed at the general practice.

General state

The experience of having gone through a major operation is an enormous and hopefully unusual event in one's life. Most people find it very tiring and often depressing. Aspects of life that were taken for granted may become mountainously difficult for a while – breathing, coughing and laughing may hurt, a drink of water a longed for luxury, standing straight and walking seemingly impossible. Privacy is lost and dignity diminished. The doctors, nurses and others around will understand and help to deal with these aspects of the road to recovery. Meanwhile, it is important for the patient and their family to know that this period of frustration and struggle is common to all following major surgery, whatever the reason for the operation, and that what may seem endless discomfort and strife is usually rewarded by complete return to effortless coping with the daily routine.

Going home after surgery

Most patients can expect to go home in seven to ten days after surgery, sometimes sooner, and if laparoscopic surgery and ERP (see above) become more prevalent this may shorten to four to seven days. By discharge they are taking a normal diet, the bowel is usually functioning satisfactorily and they are able to get about. If there is a stoma, the patient will have learned how to look after it, though they will continue to consolidate their skills at home. The nurses should have checked on the home situation prior to discharge to make sure that the family are able to cope. If the patient lives alone, especially if elderly or has a stoma, special arrangements will be made, perhaps including calls by the district nurse or the stoma care nurse, or even an initial period at a convalescent home.

Summary

Surgery remains the bedrock of modern treatment for bowel cancer and can offer cure to around 50 per cent of patients. Much goes into planning, and the techniques require a more specialized approach than in the past. We have attempted to give a very comprehensive picture of the surgical experience; next we will look at the ever expanding opportunities to improve on the results achieved by surgery alone through the use of drugs, radiotherapy and other non-surgical options.

CHAPTER

8 The role of the pathologist

Pathology is that branch of medicine concerned with the understanding and description of the processes and outcomes of disease. The pathologist plays a very important part in the decisions involved in treatment planning and in predicting the outcome once treatment has been carried out.

> **myth**
> The pathologist is the final judge – give them the evidence and they hand down the sentence.

> **fact**
> No single doctor, whatever their specialty, always gets it right. Surgeons and oncologists rely on the pathologist to come up with their special evidence to help advise the patient about further treatment, but the doctors together can only offer a guide on prognosis. The clinicians and the patient finally have to use the evidence to make treatment decisions.

Broadly, the pathologist makes an input in two main ways: **diagnosis**: confirming the nature of a tumour – whether it is benign or malignant,

diagnosis
Identification of a disease through examination and investigation.

prognosis
From the Greek meaning 'prior knowledge', it describes the attempt to predict the course and outcome of a disease, either generally or in the individual patient.

and what its behaviour is likely to be; and **prognosis**: using pathological information to give an idea of the chances of cure and of local recurrence at the site of the removed primary cancer.

Making the diagnosis

It is always best to confirm the histology of a tumour before embarking on treatment. Histology is the study of the cellular structure of tissues, both normal and in disease. Using the microscope, the pathologist is able to identify changes in the structure of cells that are characteristic of particular diseases. Further, in cancer they can tell whether the tumour is likely to be **aggressive**, and therefore one that might be more likely to grow into nearby organs, or to shed cells that can escape to travel elsewhere in the body, leading to secondary tumours. This is possible at diagnosis only if the surgeon, endoscopist or radiologist is able to take a sample from the tumour. The surgeon may do this simply by taking a biopsy of a rectal tumour via the sigmoidoscope at the outpatient visit; the endoscopist can sample the tumour if it is further back along the colon. For an area of disease outside the bowel, such as a suspected area of recurrence in the pelvis or liver, the radiologist can use an ultrasound or a CT scan to guide them as they insert a biopsy needle to retrieve a sample.

aggressive malignancy
A tumour is said to be aggressive if it spreads quickly and widely compared with other cases of the same type.

Normal cells are said to be differentiated, as they develop from the uniform appearance of the cells found in a very early embryo into different cells types which become muscle, bone, blood, brain, bowel mucosa and so on. Cancer cells look different to a variable degree from the normal tissue from which they develop, and the degree of difference is known as **differentiation** or 'histological grade'. The cells may bear almost no resemblance to normal bowel mucosal cells, in which case they are said to be poorly differentiated, or high grade. In bowel cancer, this type is in the minority. If they resemble normal cells they are said to be well differentiated, while tumour cells between these extremes are moderately differentiated. These two groups constitute the great majority of bowel cancers. The poorer the differentiation, or histological grade, the more aggressive the tumour is likely to be, and the worse the prognosis. Benign tumour cells can look like a well-differentiated cancer, so that histological confirmation of malignancy is not always possible from a superficial biopsy.

Sometimes there is a surprise down the microscope: there may be evidence that the tumour is of a rarer type, such as a carcinoid or stromal tumour and not a typical adenocarcinoma. This is very important as treatment is completely different in such cases.

> **differentiation**
> In normal tissue, this relates to alteration of appearance of a cell to reflect its function in a particular tissue, such as muscle or bowel mucosa; in cancer, it refers to the degree of resemblance of cancer cells to the normal 'parent' cells.

Assessing the prognosis

The word 'prognosis' derives from Greek, and literally means 'prior knowledge'. In this context this means predicting the likely course of a disease before events have occurred, usually at the time of diagnosis, or more particularly after full investigation, surgical treatment and pathological examination of the tissue removed.

As mentioned above, an idea of prognosis can be had from microscopic examination of any biopsies. A much firmer prediction can only be made following surgery. The pathologist dissects the specimen removed during surgery, and records the so-called **naked eye appearance** and the appearances down the microscope – the histology.

naked eye appearance
Description by the pathologist of tissue using no more than a well-trained pair of eyes.

Naked eye appearance

Before beginning dissection the pathologist records the shape, size and appearance of the primary tumour (see Plates 10(a) and (b)). The primary tumour is then cut through to allow assessment of the degree and pattern of spread of the primary tumour. How far has it grown from its origin in the mucosa? Has it penetrated through the muscle wall of the bowel and, if so, has it reached the outer surface of the specimen? Based on evidence gained during pre-operative investigation the resection may have been extended to include surrounding organs, such as part of the vagina or the bladder. The pathologist will get some idea whether those organs have been invaded, as tumour tissue is white or grey compared to the colour of the normal tissue around it.

circumferential resection margin (CRM)
Outer surface of a surgical specimen. Ideally the tumour does not extend to the CRM; if cancer is found at the CRM, there is obviously the chance that the surgeon has cut through the cancer, perhaps leaving some behind.

Spread to the outer surface of the specimen is particularly important as it may suggest the surgeon has cut through the tumour, leaving some behind. Usually this will have been unavoidable if the tumour was extensive, even with the surgeon cutting out the widest possible amount of tissue. In a rectal cancer case, this outer surface is called the **circumferential resection margin**, or CRM, and finding cancer here indicates a high risk for local recurrence. The pathologist goes on to dissect out the lymph glands in the specimen and will gain a good idea of whether they are involved (cancerous) by their size, appearance and texture. The total number of nodes, whether involved or not, is counted prior to their preparation for examination under the microscope.

> **my experience**
>
> After my operation I wanted to see what they had cut out of me. They showed me the pathologist's pictures but that somehow wasn't enough – I really wanted to 'meet' my cancer. So they took me down to pathology. Somehow seeing it there, seeing what had caused our grief, helped me to focus on the future and to be more determined to win through.

Down the microscope

Multiple samples from the primary tumour and from the lymph nodes are prepared for examination under the microscope. The pathologist is then able to report on the following important prognostic points:

✧ *Differentiation* – Sometimes the degree of cell differentiation varies in different parts of the tumour, so the small pre-operative biopsy may have 'under-read' the grade if poorly differentiated tissue is found in the operative specimen when only well or moderately differentiated tissue was all that was found in the biopsy. This immediately affects the likelihood of cure.

✧ *Local spread* – The precise degree of invasion of the tumour into the surrounding tissues, including the number of millimetres beyond the outer surface of the muscle wall, and whether any other organ(s) included are

Q If I had gone to the doctor as soon as I had my first symptom, would my tumour have been at an earlier pathological stage, so that my chances would have been better?

A The dreaded 'what if?' question. It's natural to wonder whether you could have changed things, to blame yourself or your circumstances. Dealing with the here and now must be the focus. But, as it happens, we don't think it works like that: six months, or even twelve, simply does not seem to be crucial: cancer progresses more slowly than that.

microvascular invasion
The finding of cancer cells in the microscopic veins and lymphatics close to a primary cancer – a feature associated with a worse prognosis.

involved. The pattern of the deepest margin of the tumour is prognostically important: is the edge uniform – like the spreading rings around a stone thrown into a pond – or is it broken up into fingers and islands of cancer cells (the latter carries a worse prognosis)? Are there lots of lymphocytes (the body's defence cells) around the advancing tumour edge? Good news if there are.

✧ *Spread beyond the primary tumour* – First the pathologist confirms whether there is spread into the lymph glands, and if so, how many are 'positive' (the prognosis is worse if four or more nodes contain tumour, or if the lymph gland furthest away from the tumour contains cancer). The pathologist looks for cancer cells in very small veins and lymphatics (**microvascular invasion**) as this is an unfavourable feature. The circumferential margin is examined in particular detail to check any naked eye suspicion of involvement.

Determining the pathological stage

Is the patient likely to survive the disease? How big is the risk of local recurrence? Should the patient be advised that post-operative treatment should be given? If so, should that be chemotherapy, radiotherapy or both? All these are questions that the pathologist can help with through this careful investigation. Perhaps their most pre-eminent predecessor was **Cuthbert Dukes**, who invented the first tumour staging system in the 1930s; he used pathological information to predict the percentage chance of cure for each patient, translating it into three 'stages', A, B and C (see Figure 8.1). He said that 90 per cent of Dukes' stage A patients would survive **five years**, with every likelihood of cure. This percentage fell to 60 per cent for stage B, and 30 per cent for stage C. His system required just two pieces of information:

✧ Whether the tumour has breached the muscle wall of the bowel

✧ Whether any lymph node contains tumour.

Combinations of 'yes' and 'no' for these parameters pan out as follows for the three stages:

Stage A Breached the muscle wall – no
Lymph node involvement – no
Stage B Breached muscle wall – yes
Lymph node involvement – no
Stage C Breached muscle wall – can be yes or no
Lymph node involvement – yes

Dukes made one refinement in the 1940s, dividing stage C into C1 and C2, the latter indicating when the lymph node furthest from the primary tumour contains cancer cells; this drops the chance of survival until five years to around 20 per cent.

Several variations of Dukes' system have been developed down the years, but the original has stood the test of time and is still used in many hospitals today. However, more widely used now is the **TNM system**, in which separate stages are applied to the primary tumour (T), the lymph nodes (N), and whether distant metastases are present (M). A number follows each letter, and the higher the number, the more serious the state of that element.

Cuthbert Dukes
Eminent British pathologist of the 1920s–50s, recognized world-wide for his work in bowel cancer pathology and, in particular, the invention of his pathological staging system.

five year survival
Parameter used generally to measure cancer treatment outcome. In bowel cancer, five year survival is taken as (more or less) synonymous with cure.

TNM system
Modern method of staging cancers, agreed through international collaboration, describing the stage of advance in the primary tumour (T), lymph nodes (N) and distant metastasis (M).

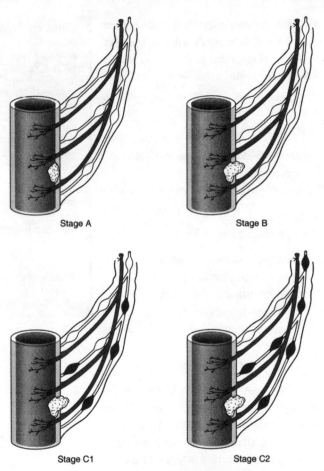

Stage A

Stage B

Stage C1

Stage C2

Figure 8.1 Dukes' pathological staging system. This is a system whereby the pathologist can predict the chance of survival for the patient after surgery. Stage A – the tumour has not spread beyond the bowel wall, and no lymph glands are involved. Stage B – the tumour has spread beyond the bowel wall, and no lymph glands are involved. Stage C – Whatever the extent of the primary tumour, lymph glands are found to be involved. If the lymph gland farthest away from the primary tumour contains cancer cells, this is stage C2, and signifies a very poor outlook. Lesser degrees of lymph gland involvement constitute stage C1, which carries a slightly better prognosis than C2.

There are refinements that will not be described here, but broadly T has four stages, N has three, and M has two:

T1   Extends into the submucosa

T2   Into the muscle layer but not through it

T3   Beyond muscle layer, either into the tissues surrounding the rectum, or to reach, but not breach, the peritoneum covering the colon

T4   Involvement of a nearby organ in either rectum or colon cancer, but at least penetrating through the peritoneum in colon cancer

N0   No lymph node involvement

N1   Cancer in one to three lymph nodes

N2   Cancer in four or more lymph nodes

M0   No distant spread

M1   Distant spread

A typical notation might be T3 N1 M0. TNM provides a more precise description than a simple Dukes' stage – for instance, Dukes' stage C includes 16 combinations of T, N and M, each with different chances of survival and risk of local recurrence. TNM certainly has advantages when comparing the results of research trials of different treatments or the results of treatment in different hospitals.

Summary

Despite best efforts, current staging systems cannot give completely reliable predictions of outcome. For instance, some patients can only be told that they have a 50 per cent chance of cure, no more useful than tossing a coin. Attempts to refine and strengthen prognostic predictions have so far not taken us much beyond Dukes. The ideal staging systems would have just two stages – cured or not cured, with 100 per cent and 0 per cent predicted survivals; this would allow further research and treatment to be directed very precisely at those with the poor prognosis.

We may move some way forward using molecular profiling, a process in which the characteristics of a tumour at the molecular level may be used to refine our prediction. Much research is going into this possibility.

CHAPTER

9

Radiotherapy and chemotherapy

Although surgery remains the main treatment in most cases of bowel cancer, radiotherapy ('XRT' for short) and chemotherapy ('chemo' for short) play an increasing role. They may be used separately or together, as **adjuvants** to surgery (additive treatment, aimed at increasing the chance of cure compared to surgery alone), or as palliative treatment for those in whom cure is not possible and for whom symptom control and enhancement of life (quality and length) are the main priorities. Before we get into detail about these increasingly powerful tools, we should first look at how we have learned what they can offer: we need to look at how clinical scientists have developed and tested these treatments.

> **adjuvant**
> In this context means 'add on' therapy, aimed at improving on the results of surgery alone in attempting the cure of cancer.

Clinical trials of new treatments

New drugs start out on the laboratory bench, with research into chemicals that might damage or kill cancer cells. Animal studies follow, checking for the drug's effects on cancer introduced into the animals and looking for any possibly harmful side effects. Just these stages can take years: it is only when a substance shows promise after going through these steps that its use in humans is even considered. Human trials are performed in three phases, known wholly appropriately as Phases I, II and III.

The Phase I Trial

In cancer research this usually involves a few patients – perhaps ten or 20 – who have an advanced stage of the target disease and who want to take part in the hunt for new treatments. In Phase I the only questions are: Is the treatment safe? What might be an appropriate dose, balancing the possibility of effectiveness against any side effects? Remember, the substance has only reached this point after very rigorous safety testing in the laboratory, including animal studies.

The Phase II Trial

Once the substance is deemed safe to proceed, the next phase, involving more patients – perhaps up to 100 – looks in greater detail at safety and predicts whether the drug might have a clinically useful anti-cancer effect.

The Phase III Trial

This is when testing begins to answer the most important question: How does the new treatment compare with the current *standard* treatment?

The scientific basis of the Phase III Trial is the comparison of the new drug versus the standard treatment in two identical populations of patients. This research method is known as the 'randomized controlled trial' (RCT), in which no one, including and especially the doctors and scientists, plays any direct part in 'choosing' treatments for individual patients: there might be an unconscious tendency, say, to give the new treatment preferentially to patients with more advanced disease, thinking it would give them 'the best chance'. This would introduce bias to the comparison, so that the new drug's true effect might be masked. The outcome is affected by many factors besides the drug – the disease stage, general health and the attitude of the medical team to the clinical situation can all affect the outcome of a particular treatment. The only way to make sure that the drug is the sole factor differing between the groups of patients is to allocate patients *randomly* to one treatment or the other, usually using a computer to make that random allocation. Then, when the characteristics of the two groups are analysed it will be found that, by the 'magic' of computer **randomization**, overall the groups are equivalent in all features – age, gender, smoking habits, weight, social class, disease stage – all, that is, except for the treatment allocated. Now, when it comes to comparing the survival of patients, the length of time before recurrence, their quality of life – or whatever seems right to test – we are more confident that we will have a reliable comparison because the *only* factor that could explain any observed difference is the treatment.

Very rigorous procedures ensure that patients know precisely what their participation involves

randomization
Process by which patients are randomly selected to receive one of the treatments available in a RCT. This increases the likelihood that the only important difference between patients in the treatment groups is the type of treatment received.

before they formally give their consent. Randomized trials only yield useful information if enough patients join in; otherwise the trial results are not so useful and cannot be relied upon in drug development. Such trials require the cooperation of hundreds or thousands of patients and very careful involvement by the doctors, nurses and trial staff over the several years that it will take to recruit the required number of patients and to follow their progress.

Trials and tribulations

It is important that the general public avoids the notion that they are being asked to be 'guinea pigs' if approached to join a randomized trial, and that their doctor ought to *know* what the 'right' treatment should be. The simple truth is that doctors and scientists are not infallible and all-knowing! The best doctors are only too aware of the shortcomings of the available treatment options, and want to advance medical knowledge by taking part, with their patients, in studies such as those described above. Of course, it would be unethical to conduct an RCT if it was already known, or there was a reason to believe, that one treatment was significantly better than the other.

my experience

I panicked when I first found out that I had colon cancer. I knew that my future depended on my doctors and I had to believe that they knew how to cure me, even that theirs were the best possible hands to be in. So it came as a shock when they said that they did not know what was the best chemotherapy to give me, and that they wanted to leave it to a computer to decide. It's still a worry for me, but I understand better now that taking part in research trials is the only way to improve treatment, and it helps me to know that my taking part will make it easier to choose treatments for other patients in the future.

So now let's look at where several decades of such scientific study have brought us in the evolution of new treatments in an age-old disease.

Radiotherapy

Radiation plays many roles in modern life – in electricity generation, in medical diagnosis and in medical treatment ('therapeutic radiation'), and as a potential weapon.

In this chapter we are talking about the therapeutic, rather than diagnostic, use of X-radiation. Other forms of radiation are also used therapeutically, but much less widely; in this category are particle emission from isotopes (unstable molecular versions of elements that shed subatomic particles that can be used as therapeutic energy source), ultraviolet light, radio waves, laser light, and ultrasound (sound beyond the audible frequency).

X-rays are a form of transmissible energy, just as are heat, light and sound. Although X-rays are used in diagnosis the doses are very small compared to those in radiotherapy. Although normal body cells can be affected by X-rays, cancer cells are particularly susceptible; cells may be killed outright or damaged enough to prevent their growth and multiplication.

How is radiotherapy delivered?

For most bowel cancer patients, **external beam irradiation** is used, in which the rays are generated by a machine outside the body. There are ways of placing energy sources inside the body, very close to the tumour, but

radiotherapy (XRT)
Use of X-rays to treat disease, almost exclusively cancer.

myth
Having radiotherapy makes you radioactive.

fact
External beam therapy – by far the most common type – certainly does not: it is simply the energy that enters the body, not any radioactive material. Sometimes isotopes are injected or radioactive needles are inserted into the body, but these have a limited period of activity, during which precautions are taken about contact with other people.

external beam irradiation
Therapeutic radiation delivered from a source outside the body, as opposed to methods which place the source within the patient (implanted radioactive needles, source inserted into a body cavity, e.g. rectum ['endocavitary irradiation']).

these play little part in bowel cancer treatment today.

The aim is to deliver the highest safe dose of energy to the tumour while minimizing the dose to the surrounding normal tissues. Originally the radiotherapist could only aim a single beam in the general direction of the tumour, just like using a powerful searchlight to see enemy aircraft at night. Lead shields were used to protect vulnerable parts of the body and the patient was tipped head down to avoid damage to the small bowel by tipping it out of the pelvis.

Evolving technology gradually allowed much more precise and safer delivery. Today the process of deciding on dosage and delivering treatment has become very sophisticated. The first step is appropriately known as 'planning' or 'simulation' in order to define the precise target area and dose of irradiation. Usually a CT scan is performed to define the exact area (**target volume**) to be treated; the physicist uses the resulting information to compute the shape and strength of the X-ray beams (see Plate 11). Today the treatment is delivered as several (two to four) beams from opposing directions, converging to deliver the *summated* dose of energy only to the tumour (normal tissue passed through by the rays gets the effect of only a single beam). Depending mainly on the treatment mode – adjuvant or palliative – the planned XRT total dose is divided into a series of daily doses. The unit of dose measurement (like litres for water) is the **gray (Gy)**. Palliative treatment may involve just one or several doses, while in major ('radical') therapy given as part of treatment combined with surgery to seek cure, there may be 20 or 25 doses ('fractions'), one each

target volume
Calculated shape and size of target cancer to ensure full dose therapy to whole primary cancer site.

gray (Gy)
Unit of radiation energy used to describe dose of therapeutic radiation.

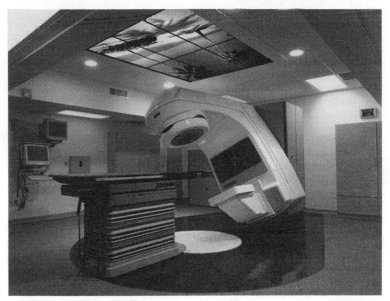

Figure 9.1 This is the standard equipment for delivery of radiotherapy today.

weekday (none at weekends) over four or five weeks.

The radiotherapy staff

There are three main groups involved:

- ✧ physicists, who are expert in the properties of X-irradiation and play a central part in the planning process
- ✧ doctors (known these days as **clinical oncologists** rather than radiotherapists, but they will answer to either title!)
- ✧ and **radiographers** who play the front line role in positioning the patient and administering the prescribed radiation dose.

clinical oncologist
Doctor who specializes in the use of radiation therapy. Previously called a 'radiotherapist', and not to be confused with a *medical* oncologist, who specializes in chemotherapy.

radiographer
Professional who manages the patient during radiotherapy, positioning them and ensuring precise delivery of the radiation dose prescribed.

The treatment environment

XRT is given in specialized units, set up in regional hospitals that treat patients from the district hospitals in their area. Clinical oncologists may visit the district hospitals to meet patients prior to their first attendance at the regional unit.

XRT units try to be as welcoming and 'user-friendly' as possible, and patients usually get to know each other as they attend daily for treatment. Treatment is given in specially constructed rooms built to avoid escape of the high energy and penetrating X-ray beams. The equipment that generates the irradiation today is usually something called a linear accelerator, or 'linac' for short (see figure 9.1). This can deliver high energy deeply and efficiently. Unlike older machines it generates the irradiation without there being a radioactive source within it, thereby improving machine safety.

Radiographers work in pairs so that the settings to deliver the treatment can be cross-checked. They position the patient very precisely within the delivery apparatus, then retreat to their protected position, remaining in voice contact with the patient, from where they control the process. In modern practice a daily dose is delivered in only 20–30 seconds.

How is XRT used?

Adjuvant therapy

The word 'adjuvant' literally means 'helping', so in this context it applies to a treatment that helps improve the patient's prospects of cure, given either before or after surgery.

Compared to two decades ago, adjuvant XRT is used much more, but this is true only for rectal cancer: the risk of damage to surrounding organs, particularly the small bowel, makes its use in colon cancer generally unacceptable.

In rectal cancer, there are broadly three modes of use:

1 Radical pre-operative therapy (also known as 'neoadjuvant therapy').

Clinical examination and highly sensitive MR scanning can give the surgeon a very reliable indication that a tumour is 'threatening the circumferential resection margin (CRM)'. In other words, if such a patient were to go directly for surgery, there would be a significant risk that the tumour might be exposed during surgical dissection. As such exposure would greatly increase the risk of local recurrence of the tumour, it has become usual practice to offer neoadjuvant therapy. In most patients there is a considerable 'kill' of cancer cells with neoadjuvant therapy, though usually some (sometimes all) cancer cells remain viable. The aim of treatment is to shrink the tumour back from the area in which the surgeon will dissect, thus decreasing the risk of leaving tumour cells behind.

The standard dose range is 40–50 Gy in daily fractions delivered over four to five weeks, followed by a six to eight week 'rest'; the latter is an important element of the treatment as cancer cells damaged by XRT continue to die during this period.

Towards the end of the rest a further MR scan is performed to gauge tumour response to

myth
Delaying surgery for three months for pre-operative treatment risks the cancer progressing.

fact
This is a real and positive investment of time for those who need this treatment. In most the tumour looks better at the end of treatment, and the pathologist can usually report seeing the positive effects of the treatment when the surgical specimen is looked at under the microscope.

neoadjuvant therapy
Adjuvant therapy given prior to radical surgery.

chemoradiotherapy
Combined treatment, in which chemo sensitizes the tumour to the effect of XRT – same XRT dose, bigger effect with added chemo.

treatment. So, from the time of the decision to use XRT, it will be around three months until surgery. Chemo is usually added to XRT in this application (**chemoradiotherapy**) as it has been shown that chemo acts as a 'radiosensitizer', increasing the vulnerability of cancer cells to a given dose of XRT.

It should be emphasized that this is a *selective* programme of treatment, offered only to those patients with more locally advanced disease. A similar regimen may be used in a patient with recurrence in the pelvis in whom it is planned to make an attempt at surgical removal.

2 **Post-operative radical therapy** This approach is used much less in the UK these days; here patients are selected for XRT after surgery if the pathologist finds that there are cancer cells at the outer edges (lateral resection margin, LRM) of the surgical specimen (see above). This finding is taken as evidence that cancer cells may have been left behind – that the surgeon may have cut *through* the cancer. So XRT is offered in anticipation that it might kill some – hopefully all – residual cancer cells. One problem with post-operative XRT is that adhesions (sticky spots, formed as a result of surgery, that cause the small bowel to get stuck in the pelvis) may hold the small bowel in the firing line during XRT; in contrast, patients having pre-operative therapy have no adhesions so that the small bowel can be protected by gravity if the patient is tipped head down during irradiation.

3 **Pre-operative 'short course' radiotherapy** This is an alternative pre-operative approach in which *all* rectal cancer

patients scheduled for radical surgery undergo XRT for just five days in the week immediately before operation, whatever the assessment, favourable or otherwise, on the clinical examination and the MR scan. The basis for this approach relies mainly on research carried out in Sweden in the 1980s and 1990s that showed that it resulted in a considerable decrease in local recurrence rates after surgery (dropping from 12 per cent to six per cent of patients). Patients receive intensive treatment – 25 Gy in five daily fractions – roughly twice the daily dose in option 1, above. Evidence for the routine use of this regimen has not been widely accepted in the UK, though a recently completed randomized trial comparing this treatment with post-operative XRT (option 2, above) showed that short course XRT was more effective in preventing subsequent local recurrence.

Palliative therapy

Patients for whom cure is not an option may benefit from XRT for palliation. Treatment might be offered in the following circumstances:

✧ a primary rectal tumour that has spread locally within the pelvis to the extent that scans show that it will not be completely removable by the surgeon

✧ local recurrence of rectal cancer has developed in the pelvis that cannot be removed surgically

✧ recurrence of rectal or colon cancer at some distant sites may be appropriate for palliative XRT. This is particularly useful in patients with pain due to bone metastases or pelvic recurrence.

Side effects

'Nothing comes for free', and XRT is no exception. As mentioned above, nearby tissues and organs may be damaged by XRT, either acutely (i.e. at the time of treatment) or later (often after several years).

Acute side effects

These occur during treatment and usually settle once it is finished. These may involve any nearby organ – the bladder, vagina, small bowel – and of course not forgetting the rectum itself. Symptoms may include:

❖ *diarrhoea* – the most common side effect, sometimes with bleeding and due to inflammation of the rectum (acute radiation proctitis). It usually responds to medication and stops when treatment finishes
❖ *haematuria (blood in the urine)* – caused by inflammation of the bladder lining and usually accompanied by frequent visits to the toilet. Aptly known as 'radiation cystitis'
❖ *vaginal soreness and bleeding* – this makes intercourse painful or impossible.

Besides local symptoms, XRT often induces tiredness, loss of appetite and nausea.

Late side effects

Side effects can persist after treatment finishes, but can also develop several years after the treatment. XRT damages the small arteries supplying an affected organ, so that over a period – short or long – the gradual onset of

ischaemia (decrease or loss of blood supply) can produce a variety of problems:

✧ *chronic radiation proctitis* – this is like the acute condition, except it is persistent. It is difficult to treat: various instillations have been tried, the most effective of which has probably been formalin, the fluid used by pathologists and biologists to preserve tissue in bottles!

✧ *chronic radiation cystitis* – besides bleeding and intermittent infection, sometimes the bladder can become shrunken, its smaller volume causing very troublesome need to pass urine frequently

✧ *small bowel scarring ('radiation enteritis')* – the affected small bowel may become narrowed, leading to obstruction, and this can be sudden and spectacular, or insidious, leading to gradual loss of function, with pain, weight loss and the features of malnutrition. Loops of bowel can stick together, and an opening ('fistula') can form between the small bowel and the bladder, vagina, skin or another piece of small bowel. Bleeding and/or perforation, leading to peritonitis, are less common complications.

Chemotherapy

The origins of modern chemotherapy lay on the European battlefields of World War I. Mustard gas, which destroyed lives principally by damaging the fragile tissues of the lungs, gave rise to the earliest drugs devised to tackle cancer. These early anti-cancer drugs offered only a crude assault on the tumour, but by the mid-twentieth century more effective, less toxic drugs were beginning to arrive. By the beginning of the twenty-first century a whole array of drugs was being developed and used, resulting from our growing understanding of how cancer cells work, and how they can be disabled and killed.

What is chemotherapy and how does it work?

Chemotherapy – 'chemo' for short – covers a wide range of medications, of which details will be given later. In some types of cancer, chemo can cure the disease in some or even many patients: leukaemia, testicular cancer and some childhood cancers are notable examples. In bowel cancer, we do not have any drugs that can cure, but there are several, well tried and tested, that can increase the chance of cure when used as adjuvant treatment (that is, when added to surgery and radiotherapy). It is usual to use two or more drugs at a time ('combination chemotherapy'). The particular drug combination, the duration and the frequency constitute the 'chemotherapy regimen' for that patient.

Chemo has one crucial advantage over surgery and radiotherapy: these latter treatments only deal with the local area of disease in the rectum or colon, whereas chemo gains access to cancer cells *wherever they may have travelled.* It works best when those cells are single or in very small, undetectable groups; then it may destroy all cancer cells, allowing cure in some who would otherwise have died if treated by surgery alone.

Chemotherapy is given **systemically**, that is it is put into the body via a vein or sometimes by

systemic therapy
Treatment that reaches the whole body, via the bloodstream (i.e. chemotherapy), compared to local therapy, which treats only the primary tumour (surgery, XRT).

mouth, so that it gets to every part of the body. Which drugs, the route of administration, the frequency and length of treatment vary widely depending on the individual clinical circumstances of the patient.

So when is it used?

In general terms, chemo may be given as follows:

✧ as adjuvant therapy after surgery for colon or rectal cancer
✧ in combination with XRT as part of neoadjuvant therapy (see page 153) prior to rectal cancer surgery
✧ as palliation for those with incurable local or distant recurrence.

Adjuvant therapy

Chemo has been used in this context for around 50 years, and this is its most important use in terms of improving the proportion of bowel cancer patients cured. In the early days choosing who might benefit was haphazard, but in the last 20 years painstaking research in different patient groups and situations has yielded a much clearer idea of who should be offered what and when.

Surprisingly a drug available since the 1960s – **5 fluorouracil (5FU)**, pronounced 'five floro-your-a-sill' – remains widely used in practice today, though others have been introduced more recently. Today 5FU is given with the vitamin folinic acid (FA) – also known as leucovorin; the mixture is known as FUFA or FU/LV for short.

Large trials performed from the 1980s onwards, comparing the outcome in patients randomly

> **5 fluorouracil (5FU)**
> A key component of bowel cancer chemo. Available for almost 50 years, and still a part of standard adjuvant therapy.

receiving or not receiving chemotherapy, have shown clear benefit with some drugs in certain patient groups, while other groups do not appear to gain from chemo. The group in whom evidence of benefit from FUFA is strongest is those with colon cancer at Dukes' stage C (where the lymph glands in the surgical specimen are found to contain tumour) without any signs of disease more distantly. In this situation the fact that the tumour is at Dukes' stage C predicts at least a 50 per cent chance that there are hidden cancer cells somewhere 'out there' that will grow into detectable recurrence later and take the life of the patient. On the other hand, it also means, of course, that 50 per cent have already been cured by the surgery. The problem remains that, immediately after surgery there is presently no way of knowing which group – the cured or not – a particular patient is in.

Trials have shown that 5FU given to Dukes' stage C patients increases the chance of cure from 50 per cent to around 57 per cent. This seven per cent improvement means that seven patients in every 100 receiving adjuvant chemotherapy – or one in 17 – will survive who would otherwise have died. While much research effort is going into developing more effective drugs, attempts to predict who will *not* benefit from presently available drugs will help us to avoid unnecessary treatment.

Neoadjuvant therapy

It has emerged that adding FUFA (and increasingly also the addition of newer drugs) to radical radiotherapy before surgery improves the extent of shrinkage of the primary tumour in many patients with locally extensive rectal cancer.

The effect appears to be because the chemo sensitizes the tumour to XRT: for a given dose of XRT, there is a bigger cancer killing effect.

In palliative treatment

In this situation the aims for chemo are twofold – improvement in symptoms, and hence quality of life, and if possible extension of good quality survival time. When it is established that a tumour, either primary or recurrent, is incurable, careful thought must be given to continuing treatment. If at the time of diagnosis the patient has no symptoms, or is at least not troubled by them, for a long time it has been usual practice to withhold chemo until such time as there are symptoms to relieve – or, as some sage doctor once said: 'Palliation should palliate'.

As new drugs have come along in recent years, randomized trials have shown that new combinations can improve survival compared to the previous standard; the average survival has almost doubled, giving most patients almost an extra year of life. For example, there is trial evidence indicating that both oxaliplatin (a platinum-based drug that has a major role in palliative therapy, and is likely to become established also in the adjuvant setting) and irinotecan (one of the newer chemo agents, established in palliative care, but not in adjuvant therapy), may increase the length of survival in metastatic disease.

How is chemo given exactly?

Most chemo for bowel cancer is given into a vein ('intravenously', 'IV'), but sometimes by mouth. Intravenous chemotherapy may be given by 'bolus' or 'infusion'. Bolus means a 'shot' of treatment, given repeatedly via a syringe over a few minutes. An infusion is given over a longer period, up to a few hours. In some situations a so-called 'continuous infusion' is used, given over a period of days or longer. In the former case the treatment may be given via a 'drip' set up just for that treatment. Sometimes, and always for continuous infusion, the treatment is given via a specially implanted tube which is usually inserted into a large vein in the neck, and is 'burrowed' under the skin from a convenient place on the upper part of the chest, a few inches below the collar bone. Two types are the Hickman and Groshong lines, which can be left in place for many months.

Chemo may be managed in the hospital's chemotherapy suite, often at the local hospital rather than at a cancer centre, which may be miles away from home for some patients. These suites are designed to offer as friendly an environment as possible. Patients settle into large and comfortable armchairs to receive their treatment. Sometimes it is necessary for the patient to be admitted to hospital to receive chemotherapy over several days, particularly if a temporary IV line is being used for each period (**cycle**) of treatment.

Adjuvant chemo courses are usually spread over six months, and drugs are given for just a few days each month, allowing the patient to get over any side effects during the intervening rest periods. In palliative chemotherapy, the pattern of treatment is more variable; infusions may be given over long periods, so long as a useful effect is seen to be occurring.

cycle
Chemo is often given for short periods, repeated over several months. One short period is called a 'cycle', while the whole treatment is a 'course'.

my experience

The idea of having chemotherapy for six months made me feel as though my treatment would never end. But it was only for a few days each month, and oddly I came to feel very dependent on those bags of chemo solution – I almost did not want it to stop as I came to realize how much it might be helping me to win through.

Chemotherapy options

As mentioned above, for decades bowel cancer chemo was a one-horse race – it was 5FU or nothing. 5FU works by interfering with DNA production, so preventing cancer cell growth and multiplication. Today there are several other important drugs in routine use, and the range is growing.

- ✧ *5FU with leucovorin* is the most widely used combination for adjuvant therapy
- ✧ *Capecitabine* is one of the newer drugs and a form of 5FU that has the advantage of being able to be given by mouth instead of injection
- ✧ *Oxaliplatin* is another drug that damages DNA to prevent cancer cells from reproducing
- ✧ *Irinotecan* is a drug that works by interfering with DNA as it prepares to copy itself during cell division.

Irinotecan and oxaliplatin were first tested in patients with metastatic cancer, and now play a central role as this context. They have also been investigated as in adjuvant therapy in research trials that have looked at their addition to standard 5FU regimens. There is good evidence that adding oxaliplatin to 5FU increases disease free survival

(DFS), that is the time for which a patient remains free of cancer recurrence compared to FUFA, particularly in Dukes' stage C patients. Data at present show no such benefit from irinotecan.

Side effects

As with radiotherapy, chemo works by interfering with cell function, and this affects normal cells as well as cancer, though to a lesser degree. Side effects are due to damage to normal tissues. They may be short or long term. Short-term problems can include:

◇ tiredness and lethargy
◇ nausea, vomiting and loss of appetite
◇ diarrhoea
◇ low blood counts (causing anaemia, increased risk of infections, and bleeding or bruising)
◇ changes to the skin and nails, mouth ulcers and rashes
◇ swelling and redness in the hands and feet.

Most of these side effects are short-lived, settling when treatment stops. Hair loss, though common with drugs for some other cancer types, is very uncommon with bowel cancer medication.

Long-term side effects usually start during treatment but continue for weeks or months. They can affect various body systems including:

◇ the nervous system – some drugs can cause direct damage to nerve fibres, producing troublesome tingling and numbness in the hands and/or feet
◇ the reproductive system – menstruation frequently stops during treatment. Infertility

Q I am so worried that my hair will fall out if I have chemo – it happened to my friend after her mastectomy.

A There's the difference. Chemo for different cancers has different side effects, and hair loss is not common with drugs used in bowel cancer patients.

occurs in both men and women and should be considered before treatment is decided upon. Sperm and eggs (ova) can be stored before treatment begins to allow in vitro fertilization (IVF) later if required

✧ other organs – the liver, lungs and heart – can be damaged by some of the drugs used in bowel cancer treatment, but these problems are rare.

As with treatment of all diseases, there is always a downside, a price that may be paid by some patients if they are to have a chance of benefiting from treatment. It is the balance of any possible benefit against the risk – and possible extent – of side effects that must be weighed when coming to decisions about treatment.

The advancing edge – monoclonal antibodies and beyond

Monoclonal antibodies

More and more, our knowledge of how cancer cells grow and multiply is being applied in drug development. A very good example is the discovery of several monoclonal antibodies (MAbs) that can fundamentally alter cancer cell growth and activity. A MAb is a protein produced artificially that identifies and becomes attached to a particular protein (antigen). In this context, MAbs compete with natural proteins such as 'growth factors' (GFs), blocking the biological effect of the GF. In cancer treatment MAbs interfere with the ability of cancer cells to grow and multiply and are designed to 'home in' and disable a particular protein (the antigen). Two examples of anti-cancer MAbs are cetuximab and bevacizumab.

myth
Chemotherapy is only used after surgery – it will never replace it.

fact
We've seen surgery replaced by chemo and/or radiotherapy in several cancers; this has already happened in anal cancer, and it will only be a matter of time before we see this in colon and rectal cancer.

Cetuximab is a molecule that neutralizes a protein called epidermal growth factor (EGF). There are growth factor receptors on the surface of cells, onto which circulating EGF can 'dock'; if this docking is successful, EGF stimulates cell growth – hence the name! Many cancer cells have increased numbers of receptors on their surface; cetuximab acts by competing with EGF molecules for those EGF receptors so that fewer are available to receive EGF molecules, thus reducing the growth potential of the cells.

Bevacizumab works in a similar way. All tissues, whether normal or cancerous, need oxygen and energy, which arrive via the bloodstream. Cancer cells actively encourage the growth of new blood vessels (a process called 'angiogenesis') to help the tumour to expand. Again a growth factor is centrally involved, this time VEGF, or 'vascular endothelial growth factor'. As with cetuximab, bevacizumab acts by competing for receptor sites, thereby interfering with the blood supply of the tumour, inhibiting its continuing growth.

These new drugs show real promise and are early examples of the translation of basic cancer research into effective treatments.

Vaccines

Vaccines have been around for a very long time. Their role is in improving the body's immune response to disease, with a track record in conquering many deadly infectious diseases. The body raises an immune response to most cancers, but this is usually too weak to prevent advancement of the disease and the death of the patient. Vaccines have been developed in several cancers and there have been early studies in bowel cancer, but there is much still to be done here.

Gene modification

The theoretical basis for gene therapy relies on replacing faulty, cancer-causing genes with healthy ones. The healthy genes are injected into the patient, being carried in harmless viruses that act like the Trojan horse; the virus carrier ('vector') infects cancer cells and replaces the faulty gene. Next time the cell comes to make the protein product of the previously faulty gene, the normal protein is produced instead, thus restoring that aspect of cell function to normal. That's the theory – there is much work to be done before it is translated into effective reality.

Summary

Radiotherapy and chemotherapy have developed from basic beginnings to their present routine role in the modern management of bowel cancer. Radiotherapy has moved forward through improved delivery technology and more accurate patient selection and targeting using modern scanning methods. Chemotherapy has taken off in the past 20 years as research into the cellular mechanisms of cancer has begun to pay dividends. In the future, their roles are likely to become still more important relative to surgery for the treatment of bowel cancer.

CHAPTER

10

After-care

For a while at least after leaving hospital the patient may be faced with a whole range of challenges – tiredness, weakness, difficulties with bowel function, stoma care, and the difficult task of getting strong enough to work and play. For some there is the prospect of six months of adjuvant chemotherapy. There may also be abiding concerns about possible cancer recurrence. If the patient knows that cure has not been possible, there is the uncertainty about the future, what symptoms may develop and when, and how they will be relieved.

Balanced against this is relief that the time in hospital for primary treatment is past. Hopefully the support of friends and family is all around, and the hospital team is available to deal with any problems that arise, and to monitor progress.

Here we are going to look at some of these issues, starting off with follow-up by the surgical team for the patient in whom potentially curative treatment has been possible.

Follow-up

When initial treatment has finished, regular checks on progress will be made by the hospital doctors – this is known as **follow-up**. Some patients will need the continuing support of a stoma care nurse, while others will need the constant availability of the palliative care team.

> **follow-up**
> Orderly process of outpatient visits to check progress after cancer treatment, including checking for recurrence.

What is follow-up?

Follow-up is a planned programme of visits to the hospital to meet up with the cancer team. Usually the visits are more frequent in the first couple of years (say, three monthly), but less frequent later on (6–12 monthly). When risk of recurrence becomes very low (around five years after surgery) the outpatient visits stop.

Why – or why not?

There is still a lot of discussion amongst doctors on the aims and usefulness of pre-planned follow-up in general, and about the various methods used. Because the whole issue is rather unclear, surgeons vary in the frequency they see patients and how intensively they investigate them. Some surgeons don't even see their patients regularly at all once they are over the surgery. So why these differences in practice? Let's look at the reasons for follow-up and why surgeons may disagree about it. The arguments for and against follow-up come down to the following issues:

Cancer recurrence

FOR – regular visits might lead to earlier diagnosis of recurrence, and increase the chance of cure.

AGAINST – when properly advised about possible symptoms, patients could simply be told to contact the hospital if any of these occur, saving many 'needless' visits. Evidence that it is beneficial to detect cancer before symptoms occur by doing regular tests is not convincing to all doctors.

Development of new ('metachronous') bowel cancers

FOR – finding adenomas and removing them prevents new cancers.

AGAINST – true, but this requires only infrequent (three to five yearly) colonoscopy, not outpatient visits every few months – and only three per cent may develop a new bowel cancer without follow-up anyway.

Dealing with any post-operative complications and problems

FOR – active hospital input allows any complications following treatment to be efficiently diagnosed and managed.

AGAINST – true, but most of these problems become apparent in the first year, so this would not justify five years of visits.

Offering reassurance

FOR – hopefully hearing all is well regularly makes many patients feel much reassured.

AGAINST – some people get very anxious in the week or two before a planned follow-up visit, so might do better if simply told to attend if they have a worry or symptoms.

Allowing surgeons to check their individual performance ('surgical audit')

FOR – the more information surgeons collect about how their patients fare, the better they can

surgical audit
Process of collection of data relating to surgical care in order to assess performance of the team, and to learn lessons to improve future care.

assess their own surgical performance, and perhaps improve upon it.

AGAINST – most surgeons do not use the opportunity to collect or to analyse these data.

How often should follow-up visits occur?

Most surgeons see their follow-up patients every three to six months during the first two years, when the risk of recurrence is at its greatest; around 80 per cent of recurrences become apparent during this period. Thereafter the visits become less frequent, perhaps once or twice a year.

How is it done?

There is enormous variation between surgeons but here are the main elements:

Clinical examination

First there will be a few questions about general health, then more specifically about bowel function, aches and pains, etc. There will be a general examination, concentrating on the abdomen. In rectal cancer patients the rectum will be reviewed by examination with the gloved index finger and with a sigmoidoscope.

Simple blood tests

A simple blood count checks for anaemia. Liver function can also be tested this way, though this is not a very sensitive test for liver recurrence.

Tumour markers

Tumour markers (see page 60) are substances released into the bloodstream which, if found in

myth
If I don't see the specialist every few months it's bound to decrease my chances.

fact
It's not as straightforward as that. The evidence that regular hospital visits and testing (rather than simply going to be seen if you get symptoms) improves your outlook is very marginal. In fact this whole area has been, and continues to be, an important one for randomized trials to compare different approaches to follow-up.

abnormal amounts, suggest that the patient may have developed recurrence or a new primary cancer. Theoretically this sounds very useful: in practice it's not so simple.

Tumour markers are produced by cancer cells; theoretically, the most useful ones would be those only produced by tumour cells and not by normal cells, so that if the substance is found in the blood it would be diagnostic of recurrence. In practice there are no 'tumour-specific' markers for bowel cancer. What we have instead are 'tumour associated' markers, produced mainly by bowel cancer cells, but to a lesser extent by other types of cancer, the diseased bowel in other, non-malignant bowel conditions and in small amounts even by perfectly normal tissue. The most widely known tumour marker in bowel cancer is carcinoembryonic antigen (see page 60) – CEA for short.

So how useful is CEA? Normally CEA is found in small amounts in the blood. The CEA level rises above normal before, or at the same time as, symptoms develop in around 75 per cent of those with recurrent tumours. One of the problems with tumour markers, however, and CEA in particular, is that the amount found in the blood is related to the volume of the tumour, so that the marker may only reach suspicious levels when the recurrent tumour is too big to be treated.

There has been a lot of research over the past 40 years into the regular measurement of CEA aimed at early diagnosis and treatment of recurrence – and still doctors are not sure whether this improves patients' prospects. Research continues; meanwhile some surgeons use the test, while most do not.

Scans and other imaging

Scans are becoming ever more useful, not just in primary diagnosis but in the diagnosis and assessment of tumour recurrence. The four scans used are:

✧ *Computed tomography (CT) scan* – This is probably the most useful test, both to look for recurrence in the symptom-free patient and in those in whom recurrence is suspected, say, as a result of a raised CEA test. It can be used to examine the whole chest, abdomen and pelvis, and is simply looking for anything that looks different from normal. So it may indicate the presence of distant metastases in the liver (the most common site) or lungs, or that a local recurrence may have grown near to the site of the original tumour.

✧ *Ultrasound (USS) scan* – This is a simpler test, mainly used to check the liver, and likely to be used in hospitals where access to CT is limited.

✧ *Magnetic resonance (MR) scan* – This is particularly useful in the patient with local recurrence in the pelvis as it gives better anatomical detail. It will help the surgeon to decide whether a recurrence is likely to be operable.

✧ *Positron emission tomography (PET) scan* – This new test, discussed in some detail in Chapter 6, has its main role in follow-up in clarifying the situation if CEA, CT or MR have suggested recurrence. It is particularly useful in checking for other sites of recurrence if CT or MR have identified an apparently isolated recurrence that might be appropriate for surgical removal if it is truly isolated.

Barium enema

This is less used these days, as colonoscopy is more sensitive, and now widely available.

Colonoscopy

This is the most sensitive way to check the lining of the bowel for new benign or malignant tumours. It also allows the surgeon to check for recurrence in the colon, beyond the reach of the short outpatient sigmoidoscope. Some surgeons, therefore, advocate a regular (usually three-yearly) colonoscopy. However, most recurrent tumours develop outside the bowel, and so are not visible by a colonoscopy.

When does follow-up stop?

Five years after primary surgery, the risk of recurrence is small enough that most surgeons cease follow-up, though some patients may be offered a colonoscopy every three to five years to check for new adenomas.

my experience To my great relief I've been given the all clear as it's five years since my operation. I always found my follow-up visits nerve-racking; in fact I found that I always got an upset tummy in the week or two before visits, making me think perhaps my cancer was back. But my friend who I met while I was in for my operation couldn't wait for her next outpatient visit because she was always so reassured to get the thumbs up. Just shows we're all different!

Looking after stomas

Modern stoma care – equipment and expert support – is a far cry from the situation facing stoma patients in bygone days. Stomas predated appliances, and it is only in the last couple of decades that specialist stoma nurses have been around; although sadly some hospitals still do not have this service.

The stoma care nurse

This important member of the team is particularly skilled in all the aspects of stoma care, from helping to choose the best spot on the abdomen before the operation, through early post-operative care and training the patient, to offering support and advice after discharge. The nurse will have shown appliances to the patient, or even arranged a visit from an **ostomist**.

Stoma appliances

There are many types and designs and they are best described by looking at what a stoma appliance has to do.

1 *It must act as a container of bowel motion.* The bag has to be big enough so that emptying need not be too frequent, yet small enough not to be an undue encumbrance. Bags vary in size for different sized people and different circumstances; in general, ileostomy bags are larger.

2 *The appliance must remain adherent.* Much work has gone into producing adhesives that are safe yet do not harm the skin. Some appliances use a sheet of a karaya gum; this

Q When will I know that I am cured, so that I can get on with my life?

A If all is well five years on from surgery you can reckon you are cured. If you need encouragement before that, there is a good rule of thumb: if all is well two years after surgery, then 80 per cent of any risk of recurrence has gone. So if you were told you had a 50 per cent chance of cure initially, at two years that has improved to 90 per cent. And if you were given an initial 90 per cent prognosis, this has improved to 98 per cent by your second surgical anniversary.

ostomist
A person with a stoma, whether it be a colostomy, ileostomy or urostomy.

is a very useful substance which, when made up as a thin sheet, forms a water-tight seal to the skin, but which is removed easily even from sore skin. Bags can either be made with a sheet of karaya built in, or the patient can attach a sheet of karaya around the stoma, with a plastic flange welded into the sheet to which a bag can be clipped. This arrangement allows the bag to be removed without taking off the karaya 'base plate', minimizing trauma. Other bags use a thin film of adhesive on a resilient paper base attached to the bag. Again this can be used with a plastic flange arrangement, or the whole appliance can be removed each time the bag needs changing.

3 *It must allow for easy disposal.* If the contents are reasonably fluid, particularly the case for an ileostomy, a clip can be removed from the bottom of the bag so that it can be emptied, either directly into the toilet or into a plastic jug.

4 *It should allow easy release of wind (flatus).* If the patient finds that wind is a problem, there are bags with a small valve to allow wind to escape without letting the fluid contents out. These valves do not always work very well; some patients find it better to use a bag without a valve and to make a few holes at the top with a pin!

5 *The bag must not smell.* This is one of the fears most often mentioned by patients before surgery. In fact it is unusual for a smell to be apparent, though even in the absence of smell some stoma patients think there is one, detectable by all and sundry. If, however, odour does occur, a simple solution is a small aerosol, easily carried in the handbag or

pocket, which can be sprayed into the bag when first attached or each time it is emptied.

6 *It should be as aesthetic as possible.* Lightweight, suitably designed bags made of coloured or patterned opaque material, ensure that present day appliances are as unobtrusive as possible.

What is it like to have a stoma?

It would be silly to pretend that life is perfectly normal with a stoma (see Figure 10.1). However, much effort has gone into making life with a stoma as close to normal as possible. In physical terms, a stoma is no bar to sports (including swimming), most types of work, sexual activity and having babies. Much more of a problem for some people are the psychological consequences associated with a change of body image, feeling 'dirty', and worries about 'people knowing'. In the early days especially, the problems may seem insurmountable – the appliance may be difficult to apply, and it may leak or come away completely in

myth

There's no getting away from it, colostomies smell, and everyone knows you have one.

fact

Not true. It may be difficult to believe, but with modern appliances and stoma care these problems are totally avoidable. When did you last think you were standing next to a stranger who you simply knew must have a colostomy?

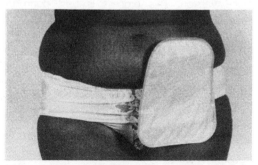

Figure 10.1 A colostomy appliance in position. This colostomy is in the most common site, the left lower abdomen. It is placed for maximum convenience for the patient, away from the umbilicus and above her usual position for the top of her underwear.

the most embarrassing of circumstances – but with perseverance and experienced aid these early problems can diminish or be resolved completely.

Bowel function with a stoma

A colostomy usually works with the same regularity as the normal bowel: in other words, the bag may well be empty for most of the time, requiring attention once or twice daily. If the bowel is more active, and this is especially likely in the early post-operative period, simple medication should slow things down.

Changing or emptying the bag

Bag changing is simplest if the base plate and the bag are separate; the old bag is simply detached and the new one clicked into place. One-piece appliances require careful removal, cleaning, drying of the skin, and application of the new appliance; the same procedure is followed every few days to change the base plate of the two-piece version. This process is best done in familiar surroundings, but most people have a small bag of essential items with them at all times to allow them to cope anywhere.

Disposal of the used bag is easiest at home; biodegradable bags are available today that can be flushed away in the lavatory. Other bags can be tied into a polythene bag (nappy disposal bags are very convenient) and thrown away with the household waste.

If the appliance has an emptying attachment at the bottom (especially with an ileostomy), it is a simple matter to empty it into the lavatory.

Irrigation

Irrigation is a very useful procedure for those who would prefer to pay as little attention as possible to a colostomy during the day. The principle is that the colon is encouraged to empty in the morning only. This means that the patient does not have to wear a normal appliance constantly: rather they can either wear a very small bag to cover the stoma or even just a small dressing or sticking plaster to protect the clothes (see Figure 10.2).

Irrigation takes about 30 minutes. A pyramidal plastic nozzle is inserted into the stoma and a pint of water is run in from a bag held high to allow it to empty by gravity. The fluid runs around the bowel and stimulates it to empty completely. The stoma care nurse may well offer to show how irrigation works; if not, it is certainly worth asking. Unfortunately it cannot be used with an ileostomy.

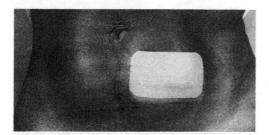

Figure 10.2 Colostomy dressing in a patient who irrigates. For those who irrigate, a conventional bag is not needed. Instead, people use a 'mini-bag', or as in this patient a simple adhesive dressing.

Stoma complications

Early post-operative problems

These are uncommon, but are more frequent after emergency operations or in obese patients. They are usually the result of technical difficulties in making the stoma. The most common are **necrosis** (death of the end of the bowel tissue used to make the stoma) and early **retraction** (separation of the bowel from the skin, with the bowel returning towards the inside of the abdomen). Both are serious. Sometimes necrosis only involves the last centimetre or two of the bowel, in which case it can be managed by careful stoma care; subsequently scarring may make the opening very tight, requiring surgical revision. If more than the last few centimetres of the bowel are dead, an urgent operation is needed to re-fashion the stoma. Complete retraction into the abdomen requires urgent reoperation, as the end of the bowel emptying into the abdominal cavity would cause peritonitis.

necrosis
Death of tissue, usually due to loss of blood supply.

retraction
Separation of the bowel from the skin, allowing the bowel to withdraw inwards.

Later complications

Sometimes problems can occur at a later date and these include:

✧ *Skin problems* – Soreness of the skin around the stoma is the most common, either because of leakage of bowel motion under the appliance, or allergy to the adhesive (though this is less common these days, with special low-allergy materials). The stoma care nurse plays a very important role here, helping the patient to identify and overcome the cause and heal the sore skin. If the cause is leakage due to one of the above problems, occasionally the surgeon may have to revise the stoma.

✧ **Prolapse** – This is where the bowel slips out through the stoma, producing a 'spout' of bowel of variable length; sometimes it can be 15 centimetres or more in length. It happens because the bowel is not sufficiently well attached to the tissues inside, so that the loose bowel can slide out. Minor degrees are fairly common and pose no great problem; a more troublesome prolapse may require reoperation.

prolapse
Movement of an organ into an abnormal position; in the case of a stoma, the bowel end protrudes abnormally through the opening in the skin.

✧ *Retraction* – This is due to technical problems. There is not enough 'slack' in the bowel, so that the bowel end, still attached to the skin, pulls the skin inwards, producing a concave deformity that makes it difficult to attach the bag satisfactorily. This is most likely to occur in obese people – the stoma may look fine when the patient is lying down, but when they stand up the abdominal wall bulges forward, without corresponding movement of the bowel. In more troublesome cases the patient will find that the bag may come off spontaneously. Expert stoma care can often overcome the difficulties posed by retraction, and reoperation may be necessary.

✧ **Stenosis** – The opening of a colostomy onto the surface is usually about two to four centimetres in diameter. Sometimes, perhaps due to early necrosis, the opening can become narrowed, so that it may be only a few millimetres in diameter – this is called stenosis. If it does not interfere with

stenosis
Narrowing of a tube or opening, often due to scarring.

function it does not matter; otherwise it is usually necessary to re-make the stoma.

hernia

Passage of an organ, such as the bowel, to lie in an abnormal position within the body. In the case of a stomal hernia, the bowel comes to lie under the skin next to a stoma.

✧ **Hernia** – The point where the bowel comes through the abdominal wall produces a weak spot, where the abdominal contents can push outwards, resulting in a hernia. This shows itself as a swelling next to or around the stoma, caused by loops of bowel under the skin, outside the muscle layer of the abdominal wall. Minor degrees of hernia are not uncommon, but a larger hernia can be uncomfortable and unsightly and can make attachment of the appliance difficult, leading to leakage. Sometimes the abdominal wall can squeeze the herniated bowel sufficiently to obstruct it or even cut off its blood supply. These are surgical emergencies, requiring urgent operation.

Reading a section like this, in which all the problems of stomas under the sun are grouped together, it must seem as though they are nothing but trouble. In fact the great majority of patients, once they have learned the tricks and gained a little experience, find that a stoma is not the dreadful ball-and-chain they may have expected.

Stoma associations

Over the last four decades, organizations have grown up, started and run by patients, which offer advice and mutual support to those with stomas. The Colostomy and Ileostomy Associations keep in touch with the latest developments in techniques and appliances, and pass on information and advice to their members in the form of regular newsletters and meetings. They play a particularly valuable role in counselling those about to have an operation involving a stoma; there is nothing like meeting a person who is well adjusted to having a stoma and who is back to a normal life, to help to strip away the mystery and fear.

my experience

I felt so alone when I woke up after the operation and realized I had a colostomy. And it didn't feel any better when kind people – who didn't have a stoma themselves! – told me how well I would cope. Then I found it really helpful to meet fellow stoma patients,who could reassure me from their personal experience that there was indeed life beyond a colostomy.

Palliative care

Around 30 per cent of bowel cancer patients are found to have incurable disease when the diagnosis is first made; in a further 25 per cent or so, the cancer recurs after what was hoped would be curative treatment.

Whenever it becomes apparent that cure is not possible, the aim of all concerned becomes the maintenance of the patient's quality primarily, and if appropriate, quantity of fulfilling life. As in no other aspect of cancer care, we see in this phase the enormous diversity – and therefore the needs – of people, both patients and their loved ones. And so, as in no other phase, a comprehensive and coordinated range of skills and personal qualities is needed from the medical team and from family and friends. Some patients find it almost impossible to accept that they are beyond cure and may resist referral to the palliative care team. In a strange way, sometimes it comes as a relief for such patients when they are finally able to 'let go', and accept the need for, and benefits of, palliative care support.

> **my experience**
>
> When I was told I needed to go into a hospice, I really thought the end had come. But I soon came to realize that the hospice gave me a new freedom at a very difficult time. I soon knew that the wonderful hospice staff had the very special ability to help me cope with my symptoms and to get back home more comfortably. I also felt more at ease knowing they were there any time I needed them.

Palliative care should be an area in which all doctors, nurses and other staff feel they have a part to play, but at the heart of this is the dedicated, in all senses, palliative care team. Palliative care arose as a distinct medical and nursing specialty only in the past few decades, and most hospitals now have a team. They aim to provide sufficient support that the patient is able to manage in whichever environment they feel best in, whether it be at home, in hospital or in a hospice; and there will be specialists available in each of these environments whose key aim is to allow the patient the freedom and dignity to spend their time to the full, whatever that may mean for each individual. The patient may move from hospital to home, to hospice and home again – easy movement to wherever is best at the time is a key aspect of 'joined up' care. The hospice, though a wonderful development in modern cancer care, is unfortunately seen by many as 'the place you go to die'. Although this may be so in some cases, the hospice should rather be seen as a haven if symptom control is not best achieved elsewhere, though always there is the option for the patient to go home to the bosom of the family if that can be achieved.

Meaningful use of precious time can best be achieved if the palliative care team can keep key symptoms under control. These include pain, nausea and vomiting.

Pain control

Most people regard pain as the most inevitable symptom of cancer, and worry that when it occurs it will be impossible to control. Neither of these observations is true. Pain certainly can be a problem for some with bowel cancer, but there are many ways of dealing with it should it occur. Pain can, of course, be one of the first symptoms of bowel cancer, but this section will confine itself to those patients with incurable disease, either at the time of first diagnosis or due to later recurrence.

Pain in the patient with advanced bowel cancer may be 'visceral' (arising in the intestine) or 'somatic' (arising in the muscles, nerves, and other tissues of the body). These two types are different in character, and are treated very differently.

Visceral pain

The most common cause of visceral pain is obstruction of the bowel. A recurrent tumour in the abdominal cavity may involve any part of the bowel, squeezing and obstructing it. The pain is colicky – a severe pain that comes and goes repeatedly – and it may be accompanied by distension of the abdomen and vomiting. After investigation to confirm the cause, the treatment is usually surgical – to remove or to bypass the area of bowel obstructed. Sometimes it is necessary to make a colostomy or ileostomy.

Somatic pain

Pain arising due to cancer involving the muscles, nerves, and bones of the pelvis or the walls of the abdomen tends to begin more insidiously and to be persistent. The most common area to develop recurrent disease of this sort is the pelvis. This produces pain in the buttocks, anal area, or the lower part of the front of the abdomen. It may be described by the patient as 'burning', 'gnawing', or 'aching'. If the tumour directly involves any nerves, the pain will radiate along the line of the nerve: thus, for instance, it may be felt down the back of the leg.

The first task for the doctor trying to help a patient with this sort of pain – if recurrent cancer has not been confirmed previously – is to seek to confirm cancer recurrence and to define the exact site by clinical examination and investigations. If a recurrent tumour is found it may be possible to take a biopsy under local or general anaesthesia. If curative surgery is not possible, chemotherapy and/or radiotherapy may be used to control symptoms. If none of these approaches is likely to help, then symptom control, preferably in the hands of the palliative care team, is the next step.

Palliative treatment of pain is likely to start with medication taken by mouth. The type of drug used will depend on the severity of the pain. It may be relieved by paracetamol or aspirin, or it may require something a bit stronger, such as dextropropoxyphene, buprenorphine or tramadol. For those patients with severe pain, the opiate drugs are available – pethidine, morphine, and diamorphine. If morphine can be given by mouth, this would be the next option, though it can be given by intramuscular or intravenous injection.

Occasionally pain in cancer patients is not satisfactorily relieved by drugs. In these circumstances it may be possible to ease symptoms using a long-lasting local anaesthetic or chemical nerve block; in very rare cases it is necessary to resort to an operation to cut the nerves transmitting the pain. Radiotherapy has an important part to play in relieving pain due to recurrent cancer, especially if it involves bones or the pelvic walls.

Cancer patients sometimes feel that they are being a nuisance if they complain of pain, or that to use medication too readily may decrease its effectiveness or make them addicted. None of these common feelings is true. It is important to be open about such symptoms and to talk through any worries about them or their treatment. The anxiety and depression borne of these problems can make them worse. The involvement of family, friends and nurses and doctors may well help to ease pain even before any drugs are prescribed. Some people have a fear of medication and would prefer other forms of treatment for their pain. Transcutaneous nerve stimulation (TENS), acupuncture, hypnosis and other methods may be preferable for them.

Nausea and vomiting

Nausea and vomiting can be due to a range of causes in the patient with advanced bowel cancer. These include:

✧ obstruction of the bowel
✧ side effects of pain killers or other medication

✧ as a feature of advanced disease, perhaps involving the liver.

Management of this often distressing problem first requires an assessment of the possible cause. Bowel obstruction may require surgery to 'bypass' an obstructed area of bowel by joining the bowel above the obstruction to another part beyond it. Drug-induced nausea should obviously be dealt with by drug withdrawal or alteration.

Nausea and vomiting as symptoms of the disease respond to a range of medications introduced over the past 20 years. They may be given as tablets, by injection into a vein or under the skin. Some act by direct action on that part of the brain that can induce vomiting, others encourage the bowel to move its contents forward more efficiently; and some act in both of these ways. Some of the more commonly used drugs are metoclopramide, prochlorperazine and ondansetron. Some anti-sickness drugs can make you drowsy.

Summary

The possible journeys for patients following the diagnosis of bowel cancer are very variable. A greater proportion than ever before are cured, and fewer than ever require a colostomy. Whatever the outcome of treatment and of the disease, everyone needs support from their family, friends, doctors, nurses and all the other professionals available today to ensure the best possible care.

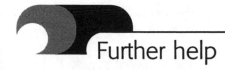

Further help

Cancer Research UK

PO Box 123,
Lincoln's Inn Field
London WC2A 3PX
Tel: 020 7242 0200 (switchboard)
Main website:
www.cancerresearchuk.org
Patient information website:
www.cancerhelp.org.uk

The world's leading independent
organization dedicated to cancer
research. Provides extensive
information on bowel cancer on its
website.

Cancer backup

3 Bath Place
Rivington Street
London EC2A 3JR
Helpline: 0808 800 1234
0207 739 2280
Website:
www.cancerbackup.org.uk

Comprehensive cancer information
available; lines manned by
specialist nurses.

Beating Bowel Cancer

39 Crown Road
Twickenham Middlesex TW1 3EJ

Tel: 0208 892 5256
Website: www.bowelcancer.org
Email: info@beatingbowelcancer.
org
Aims to raise bowel cancer
awareness and to offer support to
those affected.

The Bobby Moore Fund

Cancer Research UK
PO Box 123
61 Lincoln's Inn Fields
London WC2A 3PX
Tel: 020 7009 8881
Email: bmf@cancer.org.uk
Website: www.bobbymoorefund.org
Founded by Stephanie Moore,
Bobby's widow. Raises money for
research and promotes symptom
awareness to aid early diagnosis.

Bowel Cancer UK

7 Rickett Street
London SW6 1RU
Tel: 08708 50 60 50 (bowel
cancer advisory service – Mon–Fri
10a.m. – 4p.m.)
Tel: 020 7381 9711 (general
enquiries)
Website:
www.bowelcanceruk.org.uk
Email: info@bowelcanceruk.org.uk
General enquiries email:
admin@bowelcanceruk.org.uk

Bowel Cancer UK raises money for
research and campaigns for the
development of new treatments.
Produces leaflets and newsletters.

The Colostomy Association

15 Station Road
Reading
Berkshire RG1 1LG
Tel: 01189 391 537
Helpline: 0800 587 6744
Website:
www.colostomyassociation.org.uk

The UK support group for those
with stomas. The Colostomy
Association provides information
and support for anyone with a
colostomy.

CORE

3 St Andrews Place
Regent Park
London NW1 4LB
Website: www.corecharity.org.uk

Previously known as the Digestive
Disorders Foundation. Produces
information and leaflets on
common digestive diseases,
including bowel cancer.

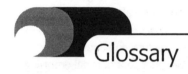

Glossary

abdominal cavity   Area within abdomen containing the intestine, liver, uterus, bladder and other abdominal organs

abdominoperineal excision of the rectum (APER)   The original radical operation for rectal cancer. Today two surgeons, working from the abdomen and perineum (area around anus and scrotum or vulva), jointly excise the rectum

adenocarcinoma   Carcinoma arising from glands (Latin 'adeno' = gland)

adenoma   Benign tumour arising in glandular lining tissue

adenoma-carcinoma sequence (ACS)   Process by which normal tissue enters the pathway to cancer, starting as a benign tumour (adenoma), which grows and then becomes malignant (carcinoma). The ACS is driven by an accumulation of gene mutations

adenomatous polyp   There are several types of polyp that can grow in the bowel, but the adenomatous polyp is the most important because of the link with cancer

adjuvant   In this context means 'add on' therapy (radiation and/or drugs), aimed at improving on the results of surgery alone in attempting the cure of cancer

aggressive malignancy A tumour is said to be aggressive if it spreads quickly and widely compared with other cases of the same type

anaemia 'Thinning' of the blood – a shortage of red blood cells – that can be due to various causes, but here is due to blood loss from the bowel sufficient that the body cannot replace it fast enough. As oxygen cannot be carried around the body efficiently enough, tiredness and shortness of breath may feature

anaesthesia From Latin, meaning 'without feeling'; comes in various forms – general, local, regional – all allowing painless surgery

anal canal 4 cm tube between rectum and anus, surrounded by sphincter muscles that control rectal emptying

anal cancer Rare cancer arising from skin of anal canal or anus (300 cases/yr in UK compared to 35,000 cases of colorectal cancer)

analgesia Means 'without pain', so analgesics are painkillers

anastomosis From Greek origins – in surgery it means joining two tubes (bowel, artery, ureter, etc.) together to restore a passage

anorectal junction Point where rectum joins anal canal

anterior resection Original name for sphincter-saving rectal resection in which the affected piece of bowel is removed and the ends joined together. First described in the 1930s, and so named to differentiate it from the old, non-radical operation in which the rectum was removed from below and behind, without significant incursion into the abdomen ('posterior resection')

anus Opening from anal canal to the outside world

apoptosis Otherwise known as 'planned cell death'. An essential bodily process by which normal cells, having performed their set task for a particular

	length of time (depending on their tissue type), die and are replaced by fresh, efficient new cells
appendix	Worm-like, blind-ending tube, several centimetres long attached to the beginning of the colon ('caecum'). Best know as site of appendicitis, and can rarely give rise to cancer
ascites	Collection of fluid in the abdominal cavity. Can be due to cancer, liver disease and occasionally heart failure
auscultation	The process of listening to the abdomen using a stethoscope. If there is bowel obstruction the usual rather dull and infrequent sounds of the fluid and gas moving along the bowel during its muscular contractions are replaced by louder, more frequent, tinkling notes as the sound bounces around – almost echoes – in the gas within the distended bowel
autonomic nervous system	System of nerves throughout the body that control many of the body's routine functions, like the beating of the heart, muscular action of the bowel, dilatation and contraction of blood vessels; these nerves cannot be 'fired' at will, so for instance, we cannot consciously alter our heart rate
average survival	Individual patients survive for different periods – if you add all the individual lengths of survival and divide by the number of patients you get the 'average' length of survival. This is something used by doctors to discuss prospects for patients, while highlighting the variability there is in survival
barium enema X-ray	The first examination that allowed anyone to see the inside of the bowel. Still going, but fading fast as colonoscopy and CT colonography (CTC) take over
benign	A tumour in which the normal cells have started to grow out of normal control, producing a lump that continues to grow, but does not have the capacity to invade locally or spread elsewhere via the bloodstream

Bethesda criteria	List of family history criteria for diagnosing HNPCC in a particular family
bevacizumab	An example of an anti-cancer monoclonal antibody (MAb)
bile	Green or brown fluid produced by the liver, and delivered into the upper intestinal tract. Contains bile acids and several waste products (bilirubin and cholesterol) for voiding in the faeces
bile acids	Substances in bile that aid digestion of fat by breaking it up into very fine globules, giving a much larger surface area for reaction with fat digesting chemicals ('enzymes')
biopsy	A sample of tissue taken surgically or with a long pair of forceps or special needle, and examined through a microscope to make a diagnosis; may be anything from a few millimetres piece to a complete lymph node or other nodule of tissue
bowel	4-6 metre muscular tube within which food is digested and the 'goodness' absorbed, and from which the remainder is expelled
bowel preparation	Shortened to 'bowel prep' by medics. Cleaning of the inside of the large bowel prior to surgery or endoscopy (to allow the best view). Methods include a strong laxative drink (Citramag or Picolax), and cleaning 'from below' using an enema (the norm for flexible sigmoidoscopy)
caecum	First part of the colon, lying in right, lower abdomen. Small bowel empties into it
cancer	Derived from the Latin word for crab. Used in a general way for this disease, whichever organ or part of the body is involved
cancer family	A family with a high incidence of certain types of cancer, e.g. bowel, due to a genetic mutation
capecitebine	One of the newer drugs, a form of 5FU (5 fluorouracil), with the advantage of being taken by mouth rather than intravenously

carcinoembryonic antigen (CEA)	The best known and most extensively investigated tumour marker associated with bowel cancer. A protein present in cells, including the bowel epithelium, that is produced in excess in various conditions; it escapes into the bloodstream and the faeces, and in excessive amounts may indicate the presence of cancer
carcinogen	Any substance that can affect the function of cells, leading to their becoming malignant
carcinoma	A more specific term for cancer referring only to those arising from the covering and lining tissues of the body ('epithelium'); derived from *karkinos*, the Greek word for crab
catheter	Soft rubber tube that can be placed in the bladder at the beginning of the operation to drain urine into a bag during and immediately after the operation
cetuximab	An example of an anti-cancer monoclonal antibody (MAb)
chemopreventive agent	Substance with capacity to prevent cancer development (i.e. one step on from chemoprotection)
chemoprotective agent	Substance that may decrease risk of cancer development
chemoradiotherapy	Combined treatment, in which chemo sensitizes the tumour to the effect of radiotherapy (XRT) – same XRT dose, bigger effect with added chemo
chemotherapy	Treatment using anti-cancer drugs to destroy cancer cells. Chemo for short
circumferential resection margin (CRM)	Outer surface of a surgical specimen. Ideally, to give best chance of cure, the tumour should not extend to the CRM. Pre-treatment scans are used to predict whether planned CRM is 'threatened', i.e. whether surgical dissection plane likely to come close to tumour. If so, XRT may be given to try to shrink tumour back from CRM prior to surgery. If cancer is found at the CRM, there is

obviously the chance that the surgeon has cut through the cancer, perhaps leaving some behind. Cancer found at the CRM by the pathologist indicates a high chance of local recurrence

clinical nurse specialist (CNS)
Until quite recently CNS only meant 'central nervous system'. In its new role this acronym describes a crucial member of the cancer team, the experienced nurse whose main responsibility is to support and inform their cancer patients – and to be easily available for guidance and help at all times. Just as with the new technologies, we cannot now manage without them!

clinical oncologist
Doctor who specializes in the use of radiation therapy. Previously called a 'radiotherapist', and not to be confused with a *medical* oncologist, who specializes in chemotherapy

colectomy
Operation to remove a part (hemicolectomy) or all (total colectomy) of the colon

coloanal anastomosis
The very lowest possible sphincter-saving operation, in which, after resection of the entire rectum, the colon – either a simple end or a colopouch – is sutured into the anal canal

colon
First and longest part of large bowel, where water is absorbed

colonoscope
A long flexible 'telescope' (endoscope) for examination of the colon and rectum

colonoscopy
A thorough examination of the inside of the colon and rectum using a colonoscope which allows not only an excellent view but also the ability to take samples ('biopsies') or remove whole polyps

colopouch
A surgical manoeuvre to try to turn narrow colon into a replacement for the more capacious rectum

colostomy
Artificial opening of the colon onto the surface of the abdomen to allow faeces to leave the body, to be collected in a bag attached to the skin around the opening. May be temporary or permanent, depending on circumstances

computerized axial tomography	Originally known as 'the CAT scan', today just simply 'the CT'. Excellent all round scan, which came a decade or two before MRI
contrast medium	The name for any fluid or gas injected into the body to help see things in X-rays (by 'contrasting' with tissues around it)
conversion	Used in laparoscopic surgery to indicate when the surgeon decides to open the abdomen, having encountered some difficulty that prevents continuation of the laparoscopic procedure
cross-sectional imaging	This has swept the field – it is taking over rapidly from most of the older imaging techniques. Allows radiologists to see inside the body as if 'cutting' it into multiple 'slices'
cruciferous vegetables	Include broccoli, Brussels sprouts and cauliflower that are high in natural fibre
CT colonography (CTC)	Computerized magic! The CT can be used to generate pictures that look just like the 3D view up a colonoscope – without invading the patient!
cycle	Chemo is often given for short periods, repeated over several months. One short period is called a 'cycle', while the whole treatment is a 'course'
deep vein thrombosis (DVT)	Formation of blood clots in the veins deep within the calves. Happens due to trauma to the veins from pressure on the operating table, spontaneous increase in tendency of blood to clot during surgery, and slowed blood flow. The clot can break away and travel to the lungs ('pulmonary embolism'); a very serious condition
defaecation	The process of emptying the rectum via the anus. Otherwise delicately known by doctors as 'evacuation' or 'moving the bowel', and colloquially known by other phrases!
diagnosis	Identification of a disease through assessment of symptoms and signs, including appropriate investigations (or after a positive screening test in a symptomless person)

dietary fibre
Indigestable food element, principally found in cereals and certain fruit and vegetables, that adds bulk to, and softens, the stool. May be lost in process of food refining

differential diagnosis
A series of two, three, four main diagnostic possibilities – the short list from which the actual illness will most likely emerge after further examination and investigation

differentiation
In healthy tissue, relates to alteration of appearance of a cell to reflect its function in a particular tissue, such as muscle or bowel mucosa; in cancer, refers to the degree of resemblance of cancer cells to the normal 'parent' cells

digital rectal examination (DRE)
Examination of the rectum and anal canal using a gloved finger – the 'educated finger'. Surgeons pride themselves on what they can tell with their finger – and it was all they had until well into the late twentieth century. It is still extremely important in helping the surgeon literally to 'get a feel' of the problem, but modern imaging is now much more revealing

diverticular disease
A very common disorder of the colon, usually the sigmoid, in which small 'bubbles' form on its outer surface, sometimes leading to complications, including abscess formation, peritonitis, and leakage of faeces into the bladder or vagina ('fistula')

DNA
Deoxyribonucleic acid. Complex molecule that builds genetic code for each individual, located in the nucleus of every cell in the body

dominant inheritance
Pattern of inheritance in which there is a 50 per cent chance that each child of an affected person will inherit the condition

double contrast barium enema X-ray
Adding air to the barium increases greatly the sensitivity of the examination to see small tumours. With old-fashioned 'single contrast' smaller tumours were sometimes lost in a sea of whiteness

Dukes, Cuthbert	Eminent British pathologist of the 1920s–50s, recognized world-wide for his work in bowel cancer pathology, and in particular the invention of his pathological staging system
Dukes' staging system	Method for applying information gathered by pathologist during examination of operative specimen to estimate of the likelihood of cure. It also assists in deciding whether post-operative chemotherapy is advisable
duodenum	First 12 cm of the bowel beyond the stomach, where important digestive juices enter from the liver and pancreas
dynamic stent	Wire mesh tube that can be passed through an obstructed bowel segment, which on 'deployment' begins to widen its calibre in order to open up the tight area, e.g. a cancer, so relieving the obstruction
dysplasia	Abnormal appearance of cells viewed under the microscope comprising changes in structure typical of benign and malignant tumours
educated finger	See digital rectal examination (DRE)
elective surgery	Surgery in which the time and place are 'elected', i.e. performed under optimum circumstances, as opposed to emergency surgery
***en bloc* removal**	Cancer surgery in which the organ of origin of the cancer and nearby organ(s) that have been invaded by the cancer are taken in one 'block' to avoid exposing the cancer and shedding malignant cells
endoscopic screening	Screening using the colonoscope or flexible sigmoidoscope in a person without symptoms
endoscopist	The doctor undertaking the endoscopy
endoscopy	endo- from the Greek *endos*, meaning 'within': hence endoscopy is any instrumental examination of the inside of the body using an endoscope (colonoscope, flexible sigmoidoscope, gastroscope etc.)

endotracheal tube	Plastic tube passed through the mouth and into the windpipe (trachea). It is held in place by a soft balloon in the trachea, and allows the anaesthetist complete control of breathing during surgery
enhanced recovery programme (ERP)	Increasingly popular post-operative regimen, which is aimed at getting the patient to recover from surgery quicker, leading to earlier discharge from hospital
EPIC study	Enormous European study tracking the health of 500,000 healthy volunteers to ascertain factors associated with cancer risk, including dietary elements, alcohol, smoking, exercise, medications, etc. Has produced supportive data for many of the assertions in Chapter 3 – What are the causes of bowel cancer?
epidural anaesthesia	Analgesic agents can be introduced into the epidural space around the spinal cord, allowing very effective pain prevention during and after surgery
external beam irradiation	Therapeutic radiation delivered from a source outside the body, as opposed to methods which place the source within the patient (such as implanted radioactive needles, where source inserted into a body cavity, e.g. rectum ('endocavitary irradiation'))
faecal occult blood test (FOBt)	A simple test to detect invisibly small amounts of blood in faeces as a sign of possible bowel cancer
faeces	Waste matter left after food is processed and water and nutrients absorbed. Sometimes called 'stool', especially by doctors and nurses, and called various things besides ... Expelled via anus
fallopian tubes	Two tubes, each running from an ovary to the uterus, whose job it is to capture released eggs, and carry them to the uterus for possible fertilisation
familial adenomatous polyposis (FAP)	Rare inherited condition, characterized by development of 100s or 1000s of adenomatous polyps in large bowel, and to a lesser extent in

the duodenum. Progression to bowel cancer by age 40 almost certain if not diagnosed and treated

fatty acids Long molecules that form the building blocks of natural dietary fats and oils

fibreoptics Very clever technology in which thousands of long glass fibres are used to transmit a picture along their length; used to make the first colonoscopes, leading to a revolution in diagnosis and treatment of bowel diseases. Pretty much replaced today by a minute camera at the end of the scope.

fistula An abnormal opening between two organs or surfaces, through which bodily fluids can leak. Examples include 'colovesical' (colon to bladder), 'rectovaginal' (rectum to vagina), 'enterocutaneous' (bowel, small or large, to skin)

five year survival Parameter used generally to measure cancer treatment outcome; normally expressed as percent proportion of patients surviving at 5 years after primary treatment. 5 year survival is taken as (more or less) synonymous with cure

flatus Polite word for gas expelled via the anus

flexible sigmoidoscope 60 cm flexible 'telescope', able to examine the large bowel from the anus to the splenic flexure

5 fluorouracil (5FU) A key component of bowel cancer chemo. Available for almost 50 years, and still a part of standard adjuvant therapy. Usually given with folinic acid (FA) (aka leucovorin)

follow-up Orderly process of outpatient clinic visits to check progress after cancer treatment, including checking for recurrence

forceps A medical instrument that can be used to take a small sample of tissue (a biopsy) for examination by the pathologist in order to make a diagnosis. Also used in a variety of other circumstances such as to assist childbirth (forceps delivery)

fore-, mid- and hindgut	Segments of GIT in the foetus, from which the mature stomach, intestine and other digestive organs grow
gastrointestinal tract (GIT)	Whole length of tube, from mouth to anus, where food is processed to provide energy and building materials for body tissues
gene	sequence of DNA required to produce a protein
gene modification	A genetic engineering technique whereby 'normal' genes can be inserted into malignant cells, using harmless viruses ('vectors') as a vehicle, to replace oncogenes (cancer-causing genes)
genetic counselling	A process of careful collection of family cancer history to plot a detailed family tree, so that detailed and understandable advice can be given to an individual and their family regarding their cancer risks and how to deal with them
gray (Gy)	Unit of radiation energy used to describe dose of therapeutic radiation
Groshong line	Implanted catheter for long-term delivery of chemo
guaiac	Chemical impregnated into FOBt card causing the blue coloration that indicates a positive test when hydrogen peroxide is dripped onto the stool specimen
haemostasis	The state of 'no bleeding'. Surgeons seek to achieve haemostasis at all times – sometimes easier said than done!
Hartmann's procedure	Old operation still used today in which a diseased area in the rectum or sigmoid colon is removed, the rectum closed off, and the end of the colon formed into a colostomy
hereditary non-polyposis colorectal cancer syndrome (HNPCC)	A dominantly inherited condition causing bowel cancer, differing from FAP as there are few, if any, benign polyps with the cancer
hernia	Passage of an organ, such as the bowel, to lie in an abnormal position within the body; examples

	include parastomal hernia, where bowel comes to lie under the skin next to a stoma, and incisional hernia, through a weakened surgical scar
Hickman line	Implanted catheter for long-term delivery of chemo
high risk group	A subgroup of a population who have in common a raised risk for a particular condition
history taking	Used medically this refers to the careful process of collecting a full picture of the development and present character of any symptoms, and getting details of the patient's general health, social habits, medical past, and any family medical history that might be relevant. Together with findings on physical examination, allows preliminary diagnosis
human papilloma viruses (HPV)	Group of virus types, some of which cause skin warts while others play a part in the causation of cancer at several sites, principally the cervix, but also the anus and throat
ileal conduit	A simple bladder replacement, in which a 15 cm piece of bowel, usually ileum, is dissected free but retaining its blood supply. The ureters are stitched to one end, while the other is brought to the skin surface as a urostomy
ileostomy	Opening made in small bowel (ileum) to allow it to drain into a bag on the abdominal surface. May be temporary or permanent, depending on circumstances
immunoassay	A test that determines the presence or absence of certain compounds (such as one occurring only in human blood cells) using specific antibodies
inflammatory bowel disease (IBD)	Persistent inflammatory conditions affecting the gastrointestinal tract, and of ill understood origin. Comprise ulcerative colitis (UC) and Crohn's disease; increased cancer risk in patients with longstanding, extensive IBD, especially UC
initiator	Substance that can start the process of cell change leading to cancer

inspection	The first of the classical four stages of abdominal examination. It means – looking! There's lots to see potentially for the well trained observer
invasion	In the context of cancer, refers to the tendency for malignant cancer cells to spread into neighbouring tissues and organs
irinotecan	One of the newer chemo agents, established in palliative care, but not yet in adjuvant therapy
irrigation	Washing the bowel through by fluids instilled into the stomach via a tube before surgery. In stomal irrigation fluids are instilled via a colostomy to wash out faeces
ischaemia	Decrease or loss of blood supply to an organ. Complete loss leads directly to tissue death, while partial loss affects function, and may also induce bleeding from the damaged internal surface of an organ such as the bowel or bladder
isotopes	Unstable molecular versions of elements that shed subatomic particles that can be used as an energy source in treatment or in scanning
jackknife position	In which the patient lies on their front and the operating table is bent in the middle, at the level of the perineum, to allow the surgeon best access to the anus. Named after an American clasp knife that has an angle between the blade and the handle when opened
laparoscopic surgery	'Lapar-' from the Greek *laparos* meaning 'flank', but used in anatomy to mean the abdomen; hence, surgery using an endoscope to view the inside of the abdomen without a large incision. Popularly known as 'keyhole surgery'
large bowel	1–1.5 metre section of GIT where 80 per cent of water is absorbed, leaving faeces for expulsion
linear accelerator ('linac')	Modern machine for delivering radiotherapy; does not contain a radioactive source, unlike previous equipment

lithotomy position — Patient lying on their back, with the legs supported on poles to allow the surgeon access to the perineum. Named after the operation of lithotomy, which for hundreds of years was used to remove bladder stones via the perineum – known sinisterly as 'cutting for stone'

loop stoma — A loop of ileum or colon is brought to the abdominal surface, opened and sutured, producing an effective temporary stoma that is easily closed at a later date when no longer needed

loose motions — Funny word, 'loose'. This just means anything other than a 'formed' motion – which means the stool is firm enough to maintain its shape

lymphatic circulation — System of fine tubes and glands found throughout the body. Some of the body's defence cells (lymphocytes) are produced in the glands. Cancer cells escaping from the primary cancer can travel in lymph vessels and settle in the lymph glands, and grow into secondary tumours

magnetic resonance imaging (MRI) — This is the technology of choice for detailed examination of a rectal cancer, involving placing the patient in a very strong magnetic field rather than using X-rays. The radiologist is able to produce highly detailed cross sectional images in three planes. These images allow precise visualisation of the shape of a rectal tumour, its extent and its anatomical relationship to surrounding tissues and organs – all of which helps to determine the most appropriate treatment(s)

malignant — A tumour in which the normal cells are growing so out of control that the resulting lump grows into ('invades') surrounding tissues, within the organ of origin, directly into surrounding organs, or indirectly by escape of malignant cells into the bloodstream so that they reach distant organs

malignant polyp	An early cancer that has arisen in an adenomatous polyp, and retain the polypoid shape
mass	Sometimes used instead of 'tumour'
mesentery	Sheet of tissue attaching small bowel and parts of the colon to back of abdominal cavity, carrying arteries and veins to the bowel from the body's main blood vessels (aorta and vena cava)
mesorectum	Bundle of fatty and fibrous tissue wrapped around the rectum, mainly at the back, containing the blood vessels, and very importantly, the lymphatic glands draining the rectum
metabolism	Bodily processes that break down food into useable substances (glucose, amino acids, etc.), and neutralize and excrete potentially harmful waste products
metastasis	Process of spread of cancer cells and the formation of secondary tumours. Also used as another word for a secondary tumour. Often shortened by doctors in conversation to 'met'
microvascular invasion	The finding of cancer cells in the microscopic veins and lymphatics close to a primary cancer, a feature associated with a worse prognosis
mismatch repair	Extraordinary example of the complexity of cell biology. Process by which mistakes in DNA manufacture are detected and repaired. Loss of this mechanism forms the basis of cancer predisposition in HNPCC
mobilization	Surgical dissection to free a structure from surrounding tissues
mobility	If on digital rectal examination a tumour can be moved easily over the underlying tissues in the pelvis, it is said to be 'freely mobile'; if it moves a bit, but does not feel so free, it is 'tethered'; and if the patient moves when you push just the tumour, it is 'fixed'. These are the ways that surgeons had to check for spread of the tumour

beyond the bowel wall and into surrounding tissues and organs until just 25 years ago, when scanners arrived, and revolutionized this aspect of cancer assessment

monoclonal antibody (MAb)
A protein produced artificially specifically to find and to fuse with a particular target protein (antigen). In this context, MAbs compete with natural proteins such as 'growth factors' (GFs), blocking the biological effect of the GF. In cancer treatment MAbs interfere with the ability of cancer cells to grow and multiply

mucosa
The tissue lining the inside of the whole GIT, in some areas producing some of the chemicals to digest food, and in others absorbing the products of digestion and water left over from the process. It also produces mucus (hence its name), which protects the mucosa and lubricates the passage of faeces

multidisciplinary team (MDT)
Another fairly new 'invention', but undoubtedly a very powerful tool in making cancer care as good as we can get it. Every professional involved in the care of any cancer patient in the NHS has to meet together every week to discuss options and check progress

mutation
An alteration in the structure of a gene, either inherited or caused during life, that may have an effect on cell function, including triggering malignancy

naked eye appearance
Description of tissue by the pathologist using no more than a well trained pair of eyes

nasogastric tube
Narrow plastic tube passed through the nose and down into the stomach through which medication or food can be injected or stomach contents removed

necrosis
Death of tissue, usually due to loss of blood supply

neoplasia
This word is from the Latin meaning 'new growth', and refers to any benign or malignant tumour

neoadjuvant therapy Adjuvant therapy (chemo and/or radiation) given prior to radical surgery

neuropathic bladder Bladder that has lost its ability to contract and squeeze out urine, due to nerve damage during surgery, or sometimes due to radiotherapy

non-radical surgery Sometimes a cancer is small enough to be treated by a 'non-radical' operation, i.e. one that removes only the primary tumour and leaves the lymph glands in place

obstruction Complete blockage of the intestine, causing sudden severe illness. The bowel upstream becomes distended, the patient has severe colicky abdominal pain, the passage of faeces and flatus stops, and vomiting may occur

oncogene An altered gene that influences other genes to cause cancer

opposing beams X-ray beams from different directions that cross at the target, summating irradiation in the target volume and keeping down the dose in normal tissues traversed by individual beams

oral laxative From the Latin *laxare*, 'to loosen'. Medication to get the bowels working, either returning to normal in constipation, or overtime in bowel preparation. 'Oral' laxatives are taken by mouth

ostomist A person with a stoma, whether it be a colostomy, ileostomy or urostomy

ovaries Two female organs located in the pelvis, about the shape and size of a flattened cherry, where eggs ('ova') are produced for reproduction

oxaliplatin A platinum-based drug that has a major role in palliative therapy, and is likely to become established also in the adjuvant setting

palliative From the Latin *palliare*, meaning literally 'to cover', 'as with a cloak'; medically it means to alleviate symptoms and suffering

palpation Careful feeling, first with the palm of the hand and then with gently probing fingertips

pathology   Medical specialty dealing with the description of the processes and outcomes of disease

patient controlled analgesia (PCA)   Very effective method of pain control where the patient 'main lines', i.e. presses a button to receive a dose of powerful analgesic. They can't overdose as a machine is totting up the total dose!

pelvic cavity   Area immediately below abdominal cavity, surrounded by bony pelvis, and mainly containing rectum, bladder and uterus

pelvic floor   Funnel-shaped sheet of muscle, known to anatomists as *levator ani*, that is spread across the bottom of the pelvis as a diaphragm, through which the rectum, vagina and urethra pass to reach 'the outside'

percussion   Tapping of the abdomen to distinguish gas from liquid and solid tissue inside – easy when you know how ...

perforation   Bursting of the bowel, leading to faecal contamination of the abdominal cavity and hence peritonitis

perineum   Area around and in front of the anus

peritoneal deposits   Nodules of tumour growing on the inner lining of the abdomen

peritoneum   Inner lining of abdominal cavity

peritonitis   Inflammation of the peritoneal lining of the abdominal cavity, usually due to leakage of pus or faeces from the bowel; may be due to rupture of a tumour in the bowel wall

phase I trial   Earliest stage drug trial in people (after rigorous safety checks in animals), seeking to test for safety and possible dose levels for further investigation

phase II trial   Next trial stage, probing safety further and looking for potential anti-cancer effects

phase III trial   Final stage, otherwise known as a randomized controlled trial (RCT), the scientific tool that compares a new treatment with the best existing

	treatment, and measures the size of any benefit from the new treatment
pneumaturia	Word used by doctors to describe air in the urine, usually due to a fistula from the bowel
polluting agents	Substances released into the environment that can have harmful effects, such as chemical waste, oil, tobacco smoke
polyp	A small lump – often on a stalk, like a cherry but sometimes a flat plaque ('sessile polyp') – growing from an epithelial surface. These can grow in several organs, including the bowel, uterus and nose
portal vein	Large vein that drains all the blood away from the bowel, and carries it to the liver
positron emission tomography (PET)	The latest scanning technique, particularly useful in hunting for distant cancer spread, and in trying to decide whether a shadow on a CT or MRI is a recurrent cancer or not
pre-operative medication (pre-med)	Medication given an hour before surgery to render the patient calm and sleepy, and to dry the secretions in the mouth and lungs, making anaesthesia safer
primary prevention	Prevention of cancer by preventing the occurrence of the disease, including the benign precursor (adenoma)
primary tumour	The original malignancy, growing in and around its organ of origin, e.g. the colon or rectum
prognosis	From the Greek meaning 'prior knowledge', it describes the attempt to predict the course and outcome of a disease, either generally or in the individual patient
prolapse	Movement of an organ into an abnormal position; in the case of a stoma, the bowel end protrudes abnormally through the opening in the skin
promoter	Substance that drives forward cellular changes towards cancer after it has been started by an initiator

prostate	Chestnut-sized organ, found only in men, lying just below the bladder. It produces some of the material that goes to make up the semen
pulmonary embolism	Serious condition in which a blood clot becomes lodged in blood vessels in the lungs, partially or completely obstructing blood flow from the heart to the lungs, with a major risk of death
radiation cystitis	Inflammation of the bladder caused as a side effect of XRT, delivered for any pelvic cancer. May result in blood in urine (haematuria), and increased frequency of urination
radiation enteritis	Inflammation of the small intestine caused as a side effect of XRT, delivered for any pelvic cancer. Various effects, including malnutrition, obstruction, fistula, peritonitis
radiation proctitis	Inflammation of the rectum caused as a side effect of XRT, delivered for any pelvic cancer. Causes diarrhoea and bleeding
radical cancer surgery	Surgery aimed at cure, requiring removal of the primary tumour and its draining lymph glands plus a small margin of normal tissue around the tumour and lymphatic tissue. The aim is to ensure removal all tumour cells
radiographer	Professional who manages the patient during radiotherapy, positioning them and ensuring precise delivery of the radiation dose prescribed. Also refers to person operating imaging equipment (CT, MR, etc.)
radiologist	Doctor who supervises imaging radiographers and interprets results
radiotherapy (XRT)	Use of X-rays to treat disease, almost exclusively cancer
randomization	Process by which patients are randomly selected to receive one of the treatments available in a RCT. Ensures that the only important difference between patients in the treatment groups is the type of treatment received

rectosigmoid junction	Point in the upper pelvic cavity where the sigmoid colon empties into the top of the rectum
rectum	Last 15 cm segment of large bowel, where faeces are stored prior to evacuation
refined diet	Range of foodstuffs produced by industrialized food industry, and including many foods in which 'refining' has removed constituents including fibre (e.g. most white bread flours)
resection	Surgical term for the complete or partial removal of a body organ
resuscitation	In the surgical context, refers to the process of treatment to replace lost fluid via an intravenous drip, injection of antibiotics if necessary, delivery of oxygen – all aimed at making the patient fitter for surgery
retraction	Acute post-operative complication of stoma construction in which separation of the bowel from the skin allows the bowel to withdraw inwards
rigid sigmoidoscope	Invented in the late nineteenth century, and still going. A simple metal tube with a light at the business end and a lens at the surgeon's end, it gives a fair view of the bowel lining up to 25 cm from the anus, well beyond the top of the rectum – a technological miracle in 1890!
screenee	The person who is the subject of a screening test
screening	The process of applying a test to a population of symptom-free people to diagnose cancer early to allow more effective treatment
secondary prevention	In the context of bowel cancer, refers to early detection and treatment of cancer or its precursor (benign adenomas)
secondary tumours	Islands of cancer totally separated from the original ('primary') tumour in the colon or rectum, arising from cancer cells that have escaped via the bloodstream or the lymphatic system, to settle and grow in distant organs, e.g. liver (most common),

	lungs, bones. Such tumours may be known as 'secondaries', 'metastases' or 'mets' for short
seminal vesicles	Two small bags at the base of the bladder where semen is stored
short course radiotherapy	As name implies, five days of treatment the week before surgery. Some believe this should be given to *all* rectal cancer patients, as opposed to selective use of long course therapy in those at increased risk for local recurrence
sigmoid colon	Last part of colon before rectum. Commonest site for colon cancer
small bowel	4 metre section of GIT where food is digested and useful materials absorbed
sphincter-saving surgery	Radical rectal cancer surgery in which the bowel ends are re-joined after removal of the cancer, allowing preservation of the anal sphincters, so that faeces can be passed through the bottom as normal
sporadic	In this context it refers to cancers not thought to have an hereditary basis, i.e. occurring apparently randomly, usually for no obvious reason
staple gun	Colloquial name for the family of instruments that allow minute metal staples to be used to join body tissues together, usually tubes, especially the bowel
statins	Drugs used principally to lower cholesterol concentrations in the bloodstream
stenosis	Narrowing of a bodily tube or opening, often due to scarring, and sometimes due to cancer
stoma	From the Greek for 'mouth', in medicine it refers to a surgically constructed artificial opening onto the surface of the body
stoma care nurse	A nurse specializing in caring for patients with, or about to have, a stoma
surgical audit	Process of collection of data relating to surgical care in order to assess performance of the team, and to learn lessons to improve future care

suture	Surgical word for 'stitch'
synchronous (Greek 'same time') **cancers**	When two or more primary cancers are found at initial diagnosis. A second tumour occurring at a later date is **metachronous** (Greek 'after-time')
systemic therapy	Treatment that reaches the whole body, via the bloodstream (i.e. chemotherapy), compared to local therapy, which treats only the primary tumour (surgery, XRT)
target volume	Calculated shape and size of target cancer to ensure full dose therapy to whole primary cancer site
tenesmus	An important symptom – the feeling of a full rectum despite having regular bowel movements. May indicate the presence of a rectal cancer
terminal colostomy	Sounds ominous, but simply refers to a colostomy where the cut end (termination) of the colon is used to make the stoma
the 'two week rule'	NHS rule requiring that all possible cancer patients are seen in hospital within two weeks of referral. It applies to all sorts of cancer, not just bowel cancer. There are also now rules now regulating the speed with which patients are investigated and treated.
TNM system	Modern method of staging cancers, agreed through international collaboration, describing the stage of advance in the primary tumour (T), lymph nodes (N) and distant metastasis (M)
total mesorectal excision (TME)	Name given to a meticulous surgical dissection of the rectum and mesorectum, aimed at removing them with great care to avoid splitting the mesorectum and potentially exposing the tumour that might have spread into it. Technique emphasized by one of the leading rectal cancer surgeons of the twentieth century, Professor Bill Heald, in contrast to previously widely used 'blunt dissection' in which the rectum was more or less pulled out of the pelvis

transanal endoscopic microsurgery (TEM)	Technique using a large calibre endoscope allowing precise excision of rectal tumours under stereoscopic vision
tumour	From Latin and simply means a lump. Although it can refer to any lump – due to inflammation, cancer, bony deformity – in modern medical parlance it is mainly used for the sort of 'tumour' we are talking about here, whether malignant or benign
tumour markers	Substances in bodily fluids, particularly blood which, if present in increased amounts, may indicate either that there is a primary cancer present or that recurrence has occurred after previous treatment. CEA is one such; different markers can be associated with one or several cancer types
tumour suppressor gene	Genes with the opposite effect to oncogenes
ultrasound scan (USS)	The earliest, cheapest and most widely available scanning method. Still very good at examining the liver for secondary spread, and the best test for checking the depth of spread of a small cancer into the wall of the rectum
ureters	Tubes that carry urine from the kidneys to the bladder
urethra	Tube from bladder through which urine leaves the body. Longer in the male as it passes through the penis
urostomy	A stoma to drain urine
uterus	7–8cm pear-shaped muscular organ within which eggs are fertilized, and the resulting foetus grows into a baby
vaccines	Anti-cancer vaccines, like others, aim to boost the body's natural defences against a target disease

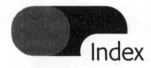 Index

Italic page numbers indicate figures not included in the text page range.

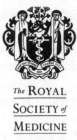

The ROYAL
SOCIETY of
MEDICINE

The Royal Society of Medicine (RSM) is an independent medical charity with a primary aim to provide continuing professional development for qualified medical and health-related professionals. The public benefits from health care professionals who have received high quality and relevant education from the RSM.

The Society celebrated its bicentenary in 2005. Each year it arranges and holds over 400 meetings for health care professionals across a wide range of medical subjects. In order to aid education and further training the Society also has the largest postgraduate medical library in Europe – based in central London together with online access to specialist databases. RSM Press, the Society's publishing arm, publishes books and journals principally aimed at the medical profession.

A number of conferences and events are held each year for the public as well as members of the Society. These include the successful 'Medicine and Me' series, designed to bring together patients, their carers and the medical profession. In addition, the RSM's Open and History of Medicine Sections arrange meetings on a regular basis which can be attended by the public.

In addition to the lectures and training provided by the RSM, members of the Society also have access to club facilities including accommodation and a restaurant. The conference and meeting facilities of the RSM were refurbished for their bicentenary and are available to the public for hire for meetings and seminars. In addition, Chandos House, a beautifully restored Georgian townhouse, designed by Robert Adam, is also now available to hire for training, receptions and weddings (as it has a civil wedding licence).

To find out more about the Royal Society of Medicine and the work it undertakes please visit www.rsm.ac.uk or call 020 7290 2991. For more information about RSM Press, please visit www.rsmpress.co.uk.